Advance Praise for *Surviving Cancer with Your Strengths*

When I was diagnosed with thyroid cancer, my first instinct was to dive into research. As an analytical thinker, I needed data—something to help me make sense of what was happening from a medical perspective. Spoiler alert: medical journals didn't have the answers I really needed. Navigating cancer turned out to be less about statistics and more about self-awareness. *Surviving Cancer with Your Strengths* is a thoughtful, insightful guide for anyone living through the chaos of a cancer diagnosis. Because no two paths are the same—and the tools to face yours are already within you.

—Jim Asplund, GALLUP® Chief Scientist, Strengths

For people who have had to face a cancer diagnosis themselves, or alongside a friend or loved one as a caregiver, nothing is more evident than the fact that every person's cancer journey is unique and should be handled in a way that is specifically designed to help them, from their treatment protocol to their specific psychosocial and emotional needs. The strength, awareness, and vulnerability that Traci showed during her own cancer journey and now shares with others through this book are invaluable tools that will help patients and caregivers as they learn to navigate through their "new normal"! We are so grateful for her presence in our lives and for what she is doing to help so many others.

—Coach Fran and Margaret McCaffery, University of Pennsylvania Men's College Basketball Coach and all-time wins leader at the University of Iowa; parents of a youth thyroid cancer survivor; and founding members of the University of Iowa's Adolescent and Young Adult Cancer Program

Treating cancer patients involves a lot more than killing cancer cells. Sir William Osler wrote, "The good physician treats the disease; the great physician treats the patient who has the disease." In addition to treating "the disease," it's important to address the physical, psychosocial, emotional, sexual, financial, spiritual, and philosophical needs of cancer patients and their families. *Surviving Cancer with Your Strengths* emphasizes this mind-body-spirit approach to healing.

—Richard L. Deming, MD, Medical Director of the MercyOne Richard Deming Cancer Center and Founder of Above + Beyond Cancer

Strengths aren't something we save on a shelf for when times are easy. Our strengths are part of us, and turning toward our natural patterns on purpose is a special sort of game-changer when we're staring down the unknown. In this treasure of a book, Traci combines her natural understanding for what makes people tick with her own powerful story. The perspective she offers becomes a vital thread stitched into the fabric of the strengths concept, elevating us all.

—Maika D. Leibbrandt, Workplace Scientist, Maika Leibbrandt Consulting

Navigating a cancer journey is difficult on so many levels, and you are always hoping that your healthcare providers and caregivers truly get to know you and your uniqueness. Here's a jumpstart to that. Getting in touch with your own talent toolkit could not happen at a more important time. This book includes affirmation and practical strategies about how each of us is wired. Traci is astute and amazing, and she is giving us a really important guidebook for these vulnerable and precarious moments.

—JerLene Mosley, Strengths & Leadership Coach

Surviving Cancer with Your Strengths is unlike any other "cancer self-help book." It takes concept and applies it to personal and practical action in a way that meets the soul and role of each person. Traci's expertise and firsthand experience make this book a tool of great healing for all those who have experienced a cancer diagnosis and for those who are supporting loved ones in the journey.

—Rosanne Liesveld, Liesveld Strengths

Surviving Cancer with Your Strengths is written in a voice that is authentic, self-disclosing, and empowering. At the same time, it relies heavily on decades of Gallup's attention to strengths, identifying them and putting them to use at work, as well as several other facets of life. Traci McCausland has been a part of Gallup's attention to strengths for several years, and she brings that wisdom to the daunting challenge of being a cancer survivor. I am not a cancer survivor, but the book taught me a lot about myself and how I might best harness my strengths when I face significant challenges in my own life. The book is not just for cancer survivors.

—Tom Krieshok, PhD, Professor Emeritus of Counseling Psychology, University of Kansas

SURVIVING CANCER

with Your

STRENGTHS

SURVIVING CANCER

with Your

STRENGTHS

Traci McCausland

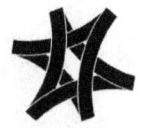

Copyright © 2025 Traci McCausland

All rights reserved. No part of this publication, either print or electronic, may be reproduced in any form or by any means without the express written permission of the publisher. Failure to comply with these terms may expose you to legal action and damages for copyright infringement. If you would like permission to use material from the book (other than for review), please contact publishing@followstrengths.com.

The book is written from my personal perspective as a breast cancer survivor. The cancer survivor stories and examples are from people primarily within my network. Therefore, every type of cancer, helpful resource, or medical challenge is not addressed within the book. In some cases, names, details, and circumstances have been changed to protect the privacy of people contributing to this publication.

This publication does not constitute medical advice, therapy, or counseling and is not intended as a substitute for those services or the advice of healthcare professionals.

Follow Your Strengths Publishing
Waterloo, IA
www.followyourstrengths.com

Library of Congress Control Number: 2025912928

ISBN 979-8-9992393-0-3 (hardcover)
ISBN 979-8-9992393-1-0 (paperback)
ISBN 979-8-9992393-2-7 (e-book)

Also available in audiobook.

Editing by Jennifer Louden | Copyediting by Ruth Bullivant | Proofreading by Eva van Emden | Cover design by Jazmin Welch | Interior design by Alex Hennig

Gallup®, CliftonStrengths®, and the 34 theme names of CliftonStrengths® are trademarks of Gallup, Inc. All rights reserved. To learn more about CliftonStrengths®, please visit www.gallupstrengthcenter.com.

Gallup®, CliftonStrengths®, and the CliftonStrengths 34 Themes of Talent are trademarks of Gallup, Inc. This publication also includes copyrighted content owned by Gallup, Inc. All Gallup intellectual property is used herein under a licensing agreement. All rights reserved. The non-Gallup® information you are receiving has not been approved and is not sanctioned or endorsed by Gallup® in any way. Opinions, views, and interpretations of CliftonStrengths are solely the beliefs of Traci McCausland, the author of this publication.

For the ease of reading this publication, each mention of a Gallup trademark is not presented with the applicable trademark notation. However, the list below provides such notification.

Gallup®	Communication®	Futuristic®	Relator®
CliftonStrengths®	Competition®	Harmony®	Responsibility®
StrengthsFinder®	Connectedness®	Ideation®	Restorative™
Achiever®	Consistency®	Includer®	Self-Assurance®
Activator®	Context®	Individualization®	Significance®
Adaptability®	Deliberative®	Input®	Strategic®
Analytical®	Developer®	Intellection®	Woo®
Arranger®	Discipline®	Learner®	
Belief®	Empathy®	Maximizer®	
Command®	Focus®	Positivity®	

To Kenny, Jay, Casey, Dad, Mom, Bear, and my incredible family and friends—thanks for the continued boost your love and encouragement provided. I felt stronger than I should have because you gave me strength. I'll remember it forever.

*To those who have heard and will hear "You have cancer,"
Look inside and find what makes you unique.
Use those insights to your advantage as you navigate cancer.
In the beautiful words of my Strengths teacher,
Curt Liesveld (1951–2015),
"Learn your strengths, love your strengths,
and live your strengths."*

Table of Contents

Introduction / 1

PART ONE: STRENGTHS, MINDSET, AND CANCER / 13
Strengths and Cancer / 15
How to Discover Your Strengths / 30
Book Structure / 34

PART TWO: 34 STRENGTHS, CANCER CONNECTIONS, CONSIDERATIONS, AND CAUTIONS / 37

Achiever / 39
Activator / 47
Adaptability / 53
Analytical / 59
Arranger / 66
Belief / 72
Command / 80
Communication / 86
Competition / 95
Connectedness / 100
Consistency / 106
Context / 115
Deliberative / 125
Developer / 131
Discipline / 136
Empathy / 146
Focus / 152

Futuristic / 157
Harmony / 165
Ideation / 172
Includer / 178
Individualization / 182
Input / 188
Intellection / 196
Learner / 203
Maximizer / 210
Positivity / 218
Relator / 225
Responsibility / 230
Restorative / 237
Self-Assurance / 243
Significance / 248
Strategic / 257
Woo / 263

PART THREE: CAREGIVER CONSIDERATIONS / 269

Introduction / 271
Achiever / 275
Activator / 276
Adaptability / 278
Analytical / 280
Arranger / 282
Belief / 284
Command / 286
Communication / 287
Competition / 289
Connectedness / 291
Consistency / 293
Context / 295
Deliberative / 297
Developer / 299
Discipline / 301
Empathy / 303
Focus / 305
Futuristic / 307
Harmony / 308
Ideation / 310
Includer / 311
Individualization / 313
Input / 314
Intellection / 316
Learner / 318
Maximizer / 320
Positivity / 322
Relator / 323
Responsibility / 325
Restorative / 327
Self-Assurance / 328
Significance / 329
Strategic / 331
Woo / 333

Resources for Surviving Cancer with Your Strengths / 335
Acknowledgments / 339
Index / 349
About the Author / 353

> You beat cancer by how you live, why you live, and in the manner in which you live.
>
> —*ESPN Anchor Stuart Scott,*
>   *appendiceal cancer survivor (1965–2015)*

Introduction

Our lives are made of a million moments: some are amazing, some mundane, and some change our entire lives. Some of the life-altering ones come on the heels of just three words:
- I love you.
- I forgive you.
- I miss you.
- You're under arrest.
- You did it!
- You got accepted!
- You're having twins!

And the dreaded . . .
- You have cancer.

Millions of people who have received a cancer diagnosis report that as they look back at their lives, they see a division: Life Before Cancer, and Life After Cancer. If this book has landed in your hands, you're in the second category and living your Life After Cancer. And by *after*, I mean *after your diagnosis*, not *after cancer is out of your body*. To be clear, you are a cancer survivor the day you are diagnosed with cancer. Period. Full stop.

You may have heard people say things like, "I'm looking forward to being a cancer survivor once I get through my surgery," or have read articles declaring, "I finished chemo and rang the bell! I'm a survivor now!" While some people still operate under the belief that you're not a cancer survivor if there is cancer in your body, I disagree and so do the National Cancer Institute and the American Cancer Society. For example, the

National Cancer Institute states, "An individual is considered a cancer survivor from the time of diagnosis through the balance of life."[1] To me, this means you are always a cancer survivor, regardless of when you're diagnosed, how long you're treated, or whether cancer never leaves your body. According to the American Cancer Society, "A cancer survivor is anyone who has ever been diagnosed with cancer no matter where they are in the course of their disease."[2] Given the vast variety of cancer treatments, timelines, and outcomes, the one thing common across every cancer survivor is the experience of being diagnosed. One day you are just you, and the next day you are a cancer survivor. The diagnosis, and not the outcome, is the clear line in the sand.

I know cancer is not a job you applied for, or a label you ever wanted, but it's part of your life now. If you have been thinking that you aren't a survivor until you meet a milestone or achieve a specific medical outcome, I encourage you to shift gears and embrace the term *cancer survivor* as a source of empowerment. I believe by calling ourselves *cancer survivors* we start to call on our natural talents, or strengths, and frame our disease with a mindset of agency and choice.

Every mention of cancer survivor, survivor, or survivorship throughout this book applies to anyone who has ever been diagnosed with cancer. Cancer is a complex and unique disease with over 100 different types. Humans are a complex and unique species with over 8 billion of us living on planet Earth. When you combine these two factors, you are left with a huge number of possibilities:

- Different types of cancer
- Different stages of the same cancer
- Different health conditions of the patient
- Different access to medical care
- Different economic status and ability to afford treatment options

---

[1] National Cancer Institute, "Cancer Survivorship." Available at: https://www.cancer.gov/about-cancer/coping/survivorship.

[2] American Cancer Society, "Survivorship: During and After Treatment." Available at: https://www.cancer.org/cancer/survivorship.html.

- Different attitudes about death and mortality
- Different personality types
- Different support systems
- Different caregiver situations
- Different age at diagnosis
- Different desire for medical interventions

Given the complexities of both cancer and humans, how would we expect two very different people to face even the identical cancer diagnosis the same, let alone the broader cancer experience? It's not to say there aren't some helpful recommendations for all cancer survivors to consider. Some examples are *rest when you're tired, be willing to ask others for help*, and *bring somebody with you to your doctors' appointments to take notes*. While some pieces of advice are helpful for everyone, there will still be many that feel generic and not applicable to you. Just as medical interventions were tailored to the type of tumors I had, I would have loved for the recommendations I read to be tailored to my personality. Rather than reading hundreds of tips to navigating cancer, it would have been great for the pointers to be geared to my personality just as shoe shopping online can be filtered by size and color. I realized early in my patient experience that one thing that's missing in the cancer conversation is considering a patient's unique strengths. I recognized this because I have a background in psychology and use Gallup's CliftonStrengths assessment to help people focus on what makes them unique. My extensive experience in this arena led me to filter all the advice, customize my approach, and intentionally put my strengths at the forefront of my cancer experience. I want to help you do the same.

This book is intended to cut through some of the generalizations and provide tailored, personalized recommendations that fit you. These will be based on who you are and how you naturally take in information, evaluate options, interact with others, and get things done. If there's no one-size-fits-all approach to performance that captures how all students learn, how all pro golfers swing, or how all actors act, then how can we expect there to be a one-size-fits-all approach to navigating a cancer diagnosis?

I don't think we can, and my own story and the stories of other survivors helps explain why. I actually never heard the three-word sentence "You have cancer." I didn't need to. I saw it on my radiologist's face, and I heard it in her voice that Friday morning. Dr. Meg Krishnan performed the ultrasound for me at the MercyOne Breast Clinic in Waterloo, Iowa, following my first mammogram. I was 39. The only writing I captured during my seven months of active treatment was frantically typed on my laptop the evening of my diagnosis and cleverly titled *The Lump*.

My Story

Today was tough. I had my appointment at the Comprehensive Breast Cancer Center at 10:30 a.m. The feelings of nervousness, anxiety, and heightened senses hit me the minute I entered the clinic. There was pink everywhere. A beautifully decorated Christmas tree, complete with pink and silver decorations and ribbons, still sat on display in the lobby this beautiful 78 degree May morning. The receptionist, Carrie, wore pretty black and pink scrubs with a collage of words including one that stood out huge to me: STRENGTH.

After changing into (you guessed it) a pink gown opened to the front, it was time for a mammogram, the first in my life. Although I was still feeling pretty certain things would be fine, I was nervous about this monster machine smashing my chest, but it wasn't a big deal at all. First-ever mammogram done, check. On to the ultrasound. Given my history of three miscarriages between having our boys, the ultrasound gel sent me back into that nervous state again. Plus, who was controlling the temp in that room? I swear it was 55 degrees. My body was shaking, part fear, part cold. My husband, Kent, joined me for this part and sat in the dim room in his dark business suit, making small talk with the sonographer, Sara; more small talk than is typical for my Kenny.

When Sara finished up, she explained that Dr. Meg would be in to do some of her own ultrasound imaging as she likes to check for herself too. I recognized Dr. Meg as a Happy Time daycare mom I often see picking up our kiddos after work. Her familiarity put me at ease. She grabbed the wand, and as I lay on my side, my anxiety sharpened and I felt a stab of fear. She was looking for a long time. Not that I had a benchmark for comparison, but this felt like a long time to me. She asked me to turn to the screen so she could explain to me what she was noticing.

Kenny joined me as Dr. Meg explained that the spots on my breast were gray and different from the fibrous tissue around them. She pointed out a cyst, showed us one lymph node spot that was concerning, and told us she'd like to proceed with a biopsy and that we would have results on Monday.

Then Kent asked the game-changing question, "Dr. Meg, given your experience seeing so many of these, combined with Traci's age, what are we looking at here? If you had to give a percentage . . . that she has breast cancer," he trailed off. I was shocked and relieved at the boldness of his question, and it was precisely this moment when my life shifted. Dr. Meg placed her hands on me, one on my shoulder and one on my forearm. She said, "You came to me for a true and honest opinion. In my opinion, I would have to say that I am 95% certain on this." Tears filled my eyes as she continued, "This is why we move forward with the biopsy and testing. I so hope I am proven wrong." If there is an award for delivering the "You have cancer" news to a patient with empathy, Dr. Meg wins.

The biopsy sucked, despite lots of loving and supportive chatter from the nurses. There must be a secret code the care staff uses between the ultrasound and biopsy to communicate, *We got a hot one here.* That, or my intermittent tears were the giveaway. Regardless, I was so appreciative of the kindness and sincerity of the women involved in the biopsy procedure.

After injections in three spots, two on my breast and one in my lymph node, in addition to this painful punching device that injects a marker into the area of concern, we were finally done.

Dr. Meg asked, "Traci, may I pray for you?" I smiled and said, "Sure." I assumed she meant at home, tonight. But she meant right then and there, as I lay on the table tired and somewhat in shock. (I later connected the dots that MercyOne is part of Trinity Health, one of the largest Catholic not-for-profit health systems.)

She prayed, and the care team and Kenny laid their hands on my body. It was a lovely prayer, and quite long and intense. I remember she used words like *benign, wash over, support,* and even threw in something about "Be beside them if they spend too much time Googling this weekend, and keep them away from the path of fear, sadness, and being scared." Tears streamed down my face. I felt so much love and support from all the hands on me, I really did, sad as I was in that moment.

They explained we would come back in on Monday morning to review my results, and likely set a game plan moving forward. I said I was leading a workshop at American College Testing (ACT), and the appointment was going to have to wait until the afternoon. My decision to keep my work commitment as planned made me feel like I had some level of control over the cancer that was about to disrupt my life.

Kent and I made sure we were on the same page about not telling the kids yet and going ahead with our plan for the afternoon. Then we parted ways to head home, having driven separately. I called my mom, and her first word was "Wow." Ironically, it was also the first word I said to myself when Dr. Meg gave me the news. I said, "Yeah, I know . . . But Angela would have taken this day in a heartbeat," and wept. Angela, our friend and Kent's colleague, had died the previous December, five months ago. Given the choice of a fatal brain aneurysm at 34 or a likely breast cancer diagnosis at 39, I knew she would have done anything to have a day like I was having. I felt her with me, her playful grin saying, "Okay, so you probably have breast cancer. Now go hug your kids, have an awesome Mother's Day, and move forward."

In between standing in the hospital parking lot Friday and returning Monday afternoon, Kent and I kept living. I called my younger sister, Kari, who works in intensive care at Children's Mercy in Kansas City. I told her about the appointment and that it was probably breast cancer, and she let out a wailing cry that I had never heard from her before or since. With her raw emotion, combined with her empathetic heart and beautiful words, she gave me permission to truly feel that it was okay to be sad right now.

Next, I drove away to a jewelry store across the street to get my watch fixed, although it was kind of a bizarre feeling to be running errands with this invisible secret inside. Kent and I stuck with our original plan of dropping the boys off with my parents in Iowa Falls, a nice midway point, so we could spend our evening in Des Moines looking for vintage basketball court flooring from an old high school gym. It now frames our TV downstairs in the sports room and is pretty darn cool.

After hearing I probably had cancer, Kent and I decided right away *Life goes on*. We could have hunkered down at home crying and processing, which would have been totally fine too. Instead, I think we both knew that our life-changing morning was just the beginning of many more appointments, decisions, and emotions to come. We even joked we could get hit by a car on our way to Des Moines, so let's not let this probable cancer diagnosis put a halt to everything else going on in our lives.

We spent the weekend sharing the update with our family members and close inner circle of friends locally that we could tell in person. We even had friends join us for pizza on the porch on Mother's Day, while celebrating with my parents. I made the deliberate decision to be with friends and family during the long weekend of waiting rather than being alone, as people are a source of energy for me. Monday morning, I drove 70 miles to facilitate a Discover Your Strengths workshop with ACT, an outstanding client of my business. Although I felt a bit like a teenager hiding a tattoo from their parents, I still delivered a solid workshop for the 20+ people in the room. Retaining control of my work schedule before cancer flipped it on its head felt empowering to me, and it was a small win right out of the gates as a cancer survivor. I drove another

70 miles back to the Breast Clinic, where Kent joined me for the unveiling of my results. Hearing my official diagnosis of Stage 2b breast cancer, including cancer in the suspicious lymph node, felt more like a formality to me than an emotional experience. I didn't even cry in the small office at the hospital when they delivered the news and next steps.

Within two days of my diagnosis, we made the decision that I would seek my treatment from the University of Iowa Health Care (UIHC) in Iowa City rather than locally. My first oncology appointment was confirmed for the following week, and in the meantime, I read about the likely road ahead and reached out to a friend of a friend to learn about her experience of having breast cancer—twice.

Through these online searches and the early process of sharing my diagnosis with close friends, my identity began feeling cloudy and unclear. It didn't take long before I was picking up on this new cancer language and was struck by expressions such as *fight like he*l* or *you've got this*. I kept seeing combative words like *warrior, fighter, battle,* and *strong*. We see that language plastered on nearly every cancer fundraising campaign.

While I completely understood people's good intentions with their fighting metaphors to fire cancer survivors up, for me those words fell flat. In my nearly 40 years on the planet, I don't think friends and family would ever have described me as *strong, tough,* or a *fighter*. In fact, this was my very first Google search after we decided to receive treatment at UIHC:

What if fighting cancer does not resonate with me?

It wasn't that I didn't want to beat cancer. I did. I wanted all the tumors out of my body as soon as possible and wanted to have the best care team in my corner. I just didn't want to force myself into a different, unfamiliar identity while grappling with this new layer of myself as a cancer survivor. Picture your daily to-do list. Who has room for "beat cancer" on there? Some days are a win for me if I make dinner from scratch or get the recycling to the curb. I remember hearing the projected timelines for treatment and thinking sarcastically, "Sure, why don't you add 'fight cancer' to my list for the next 200 days?" I had this sinking feeling in my gut that while I didn't want to disappoint my supporters, I couldn't magically transform into an American Gladiator overnight. I remember feeling stressed out and worried that my "army" of family, friends, and supporters might be let down or disappointed if I wasn't kicking cancer's a*s on the daily. (Sidebar: When did people decide cancer has a butt? It's so weird.)

My Google search—*What if fighting cancer does not resonate with me?*—led to an article on *Huffington Post* where Stephanie Sliekers states, "You know what alternative to these metaphors I appreciate? Cure. Treat. Prevent. Support. Help. These words are less anger-inducing and aggressive and place the focus where it belongs—on science, research, healthcare and patient supports."[3] Ahhh, now those are words I can get with. This insight made me feel so understood. My mind calmed as I exhaled, and I felt less alone and so relieved that I didn't need to armor up.

Shortly after my diagnosis, I read another powerful opinion article that resonated with me: "Why Cancer Is not a War, Fight, or Battle." Xeni Jardin wrote, "I grew up hearing cancer described as combat, something you 'beat' if you've got enough 'fight' in you. President Richard Nixon declared war on cancer when I was a baby. Military metaphors were familiar, but they stopped making sense when the war was me. My own body."[4] Amen, sister. I had enough on my plate between growing my business and being a mom of two boys, nine and four at the time. I felt exhausted by the thought of "armoring up" to "fight" this invisible disease I knew very little about.

Although I felt comforted that I wasn't the only person struggling with the "fighting" aspect of cancer by these articles from strangers online, I still felt something was missing. It was like when your family loads the trunk full of suitcases and supplies, hops in, and is ready for an exciting week of vacation. A lot of preparation, planning, and packing has led up to this point, and everything feels ready to go, but you have a nagging

---

3   Stephanie Sliekers, *HuffPost* (September 17, 2013) "Your Cancer Metaphors Don't Comfort Me." Available at: https://www.huffpost.com/entry/cancer-metaphors_b_3846353.

4   Xeni Jardin, CNN (July 21, 2017) "Why Cancer Is not a War, Fight, or Battle." Available at: https://www.cnn.com/2017/07/21/opinions/cancer-is-not-a-war-jardin-opinion/index.html.

sense that something is missing. You wonder if you left the curling iron plugged in, or if you remembered to lock the front door. That's how I felt. I was very confident in our treatment decision and blown away by the love and support from those near me. In fact, I would have graded the experience an A+ at that point, but there was just one . . . thing . . . missing. A question cycled through my head over and over again, "What am I supposed to DO with this?" Slowly, I realized the nagging feeling in my gut was telling me I should use this adversity to help other people. But how? I couldn't back out of the driveway until I knew that.

While my soul was pondering the missing piece of my cancer plan—how I could use it to help others—I continued receiving caring advice and sentiments from those around me. Ones that kept appearing were:

- "Do what feels right to you."
- "You don't have to handle this like anybody else."
- "Make this journey your own."

Then, on about Day 10 after my diagnosis, I was sitting in my comfortable chair in my home office when my gaze landed on my bookcase. A group of titles, all Gallup books, caught my attention. *StrengthsFinder 2.0. Strengths Based Leadership. Strengths Based Parenting. Strengths Based Selling. Living Your Strengths. Teach with Your Strengths.*

I wondered, "Where is the book telling me how to survive cancer with my strengths?"

If people were successfully managing, leading, selling, parenting, and teaching based on their individual strengths, then it seemed logical they could navigate cancer with them as well. I stared more closely at all the books, rereading the titles again and again. In my mind's eye, there was a gap where the book I needed to read should have been. That was the moment I understood the answer to the nagging question. It hit me. "If this book doesn't exist, I'm going to write it." My eyes widened as I thought about how approaching a healthcare crisis and the science of strengths could be connected. It made me wonder if maybe this strengths drum I had been beating could help me in the biggest crisis of my life—and help others with their cancer experience too.

Introduction

By uncovering some purpose in this cancer chaos, the confused chatter in my mind quickly turned to confidence. "Of course everyone would respond to a cancer diagnosis uniquely. There may actually be purpose hidden in my struggle." This was the exact moment of clarity that led me to exhale and back out of the driveway, so to speak. Given that my work leverages the Gallup Organization's tools and assessments for leadership development and team building, I knew that my quickest pathway to success was through the lens of my natural talents and strengths. As Strengths practitioners, we teach people to be authentic, to be the best versions of themselves through the lens of their talents. As my Strengths teacher, Curt Liesveld, shared while teaching a group of coaches in Japan, "Learn your strengths, love your strengths, and live your strengths."[5] Pitting me against some monster opponent like cancer is not the way to get the best of me. I understood that the best way for me to keep my tank as full as possible was to think, feel, and behave authentically, especially through cancer.

To test my theory, I challenged myself to put my deep knowledge around strengths to work through my cancer experience. The book includes examples of intentional actions I took that helped me feel strong during a time in my life when I was physically the weakest. It also includes advice and stories from the experiences of other cancer survivors around the world. Their varied actions and approaches further validate how there's often not a single right way of doing things. As you read this book, you will feel more confident, resilient, and hopeful. You will feel empowered and equipped to approach your cancer experience uniquely, in a way that feels natural and authentic to you.

You may consider assessments and team building exercises cheesy, a waste of time, or not helpful when facing cancer. While I know my tumors didn't care that I was using my strengths as a competitive advantage, I am also certain that my mindset and energy improved because I

---

5 Jeremy Pietrocini and Benjamin Erikson-Farr, Gallup Clifton Strengths (June 23, 2015) "Learn, Love, Live: The Journey of Strengths." Available at: https://www.gallup.com/cliftonstrengths/en/251093/learn-love-live-journey-strengths.aspx.

was. There are so many beautiful quotes related to challenge, adversity, and even cancer. My absolute favorite is from ESPN Anchor Stuart Scott, an appendiceal cancer survivor, who passed away at the age of 49. I love it so much I put it at the front of this book.

> When you die, it does not mean that you lose to cancer. You beat cancer by how you live, why you live, and in the manner in which you live.[6]

On that note, can we all agree to stop saying that anyone "lost their battle with cancer?" Nobody says, "She lost her battle with her heart" after somebody has a heart attack, or "He lost his battle with obesity," or "They lost their battle with blood pressure." We need to stop.

Maybe we can "beat cancer," the most common rallying cry, in our own ways and on our own terms. I'm pretty sure we can—because both Stuart and I already did.

---

6   Stuart Scott, V Foundation (2014) Available at: https://www.v.org/story/when-you-die-it-does-not-mean-that-you-lose-to-cancer-stuart-scott/.

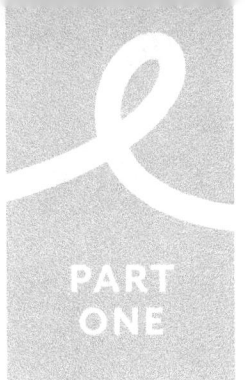

PART ONE

STRENGTHS, MINDSET, AND CANCER

> What will happen when we start to think about what is right with people instead of fixating on what is wrong with them?
>
> —*Dr. Donald Clifton, father of strengths-based psychology and inventor of the CliftonStrengths assessment*

Strengths and Cancer

You may be wondering what the connection is between having cancer and understanding your strengths. It's a fair question and one I thought about for years while sporadically drafting this book. Having a cancer diagnosis can feel completely overwhelming and like it's you against this big, bad, awful disease. So, to even entertain the idea that cancer cares about your uniqueness is somewhat laughable. To be clear, it doesn't. But that doesn't mean that your uniqueness can't play a significant role in how you approach your cancer diagnosis. In fact, I think it's a smart, efficient, and effective strategy regardless of your type of cancer or prognosis. Here's some background on why.

The History of Strengths

Decades ago, the Gallup Organization, and more specifically Dr. Donald Clifton, broke with traditional approaches in psychology that looked for issues and problems in people and began studying the good things instead. Don was the CEO of Gallup and known for saying, "What will happen when we start to think about what is right with people instead of fixating on what is wrong with them?"[7] He was an Army Air Force navigator and flew B-24s in World War II, which earned him the Distinguished Flying Cross for heroism. Don's son and former CEO of Gallup Jim Clifton has stood on stages around the world and shared, "Dad

---

7   Cathy Deweese, Gallup CliftonStrengths (October 17, 2018) "Learning About CliftonStrengths from Don Clifton Himself." Available at: https://www.gallup.com/cliftonstrengths/en/249602/learning-cliftonstrengths-don-clifton.aspx.

returned home and had seen enough war and destruction. He wanted to spend the rest of his life doing good for humankind."

Don pursued doctoral studies in educational psychology at the University of Nebraska. I've heard an inspiring story about him told multiple times by a variety of Gallup associates. They say that Don was staring at the psychology section in the campus library. Apparently, he turned to a librarian and asked, "Where are the books about what is right with people?" to which the response was "Well, those haven't been written yet."[8] Gallup associates also share that if you were traveling on work trips with Don, he would drive slowly past cemeteries. He would turn to his colleagues and express disappointment along the lines of how many people go to their graves without really knowing their strengths. He had a relentless fascination with the uniqueness of people, and their potential, and he committed his life to helping them see it too.

Dr. Clifton and Gallup went on to do tremendous research around the most successful team members in organizations. They interviewed millions of people across industries and occupations to see if there was a common denominator that the best all possessed. This research led to their big discovery that "there is no one way to lead"[9] and to the creation of their strengths-based framework, which ultimately identified 34 Talent Themes. Dr. Clifton used this extensive research on talent to create the CliftonStrengths assessment, formerly known as StrengthsFinder, which is a series of 200 questions available in more than 25 languages. A few of the 34 strengths include Competition, Empathy, and Analytical, which are common words we generally understand. But the framework also includes strengths with rarer names like Individualization, Intellection, and a fun one called Woo, which stands for "winning others over." In the bestselling 2008 book *Strengths Based Leadership*,[10] Gallup first introduced the concept of the four domains of leadership. The four domains

---

8   Gallup CliftonStrengths, "The History of CliftonStrengths." Available at: https://www.gallup.com/cliftonstrengths/en/253754/history-cliftonstrengths.aspx.
9   Described in *StrengthsFinder 2.0*. 2007. Gallup Press.
10 https://www.followyourstrengths.com/book.

are a helpful way to categorize the 34 strengths at a higher level and include the following:
- Executing: How you make things happen
- Influencing: How you influence others
- Relationship Building: How you build and nurture strong relationships
- Strategic Thinking: How you absorb, think about, and analyze information and situations

Executing	Influencing	Relationship Building	Strategic Thinking
People with dominant Executing themes know how to **make things happen.**	People with dominant Influencing themes know how to **take charge, speak up, and make sure the team is heard.**	People with dominant Relationship Building themes have the ability to build strong relationships that can **hold a team together and make the team greater than the sum of its parts.**	People with dominant Strategic Thinking themes help teams consider what could be. **They absorb and analyze information that can inform better decisions.**
Achiever Arranger Belief Consistency Deliberative Discipline Focus Responsibility Restorative	Activator Command Communication Competition Maximizer Self-Assurance Significance Woo	Adaptability Connectedness Developer Empathy Harmony Includer Individualization Positivity Relator	Analytical Context Futuristic Ideation Input Intellection Learner Strategic

I've heard Gallup associates who worked with Don in the 1990s say that he would walk around the office holding a stack of note cards, one for each strength. He would ask people to do their own manual card sort and share his vision of how incredible it would be if they could get one million people to learn their strengths. To date, the CliftonStrengths assessment has been taken by over 35 million people around the world. Jim Clifton says, "The results are the most unusual in the world—they determine what's right with you. There was never a tool like this until Gallup invented one. When you make the most of your strengths, there are no limits to what you can do."[11] Shortly before his passing from metastasized esophageal cancer in 2003, Dr. Clifton received the American Psychological Association's Presidential Commendation as the Father of Strengths-Based Psychology and the Grandfather of Positive Psychology.

The Power of Strengths

So, how does this have anything to do with cancer? Well, judging solely by the outcomes data of Gallup, it could have a lot to do with how you feel while you endure a cancer diagnosis. Gallup's data shows that people who have the opportunity to use their strengths are:

3x	6x	6x
as likely to report having an excellent quality of life	as likely to strongly agree that they have the chance to do what they do best every day	as likely to be engaged in their job

Further research by Gallup shows that:

> ... using strengths leads to improved health and wellness outcomes. The more hours each day that Americans can use their strengths to do what they do best, the less likely they are to

---

11 "Discover Your CliftonStrengths" (2007) *StrengthsFinder 2.0*. Gallup Press.

report experiencing worry, stress, anger, sadness, or physical pain during the previous day. The more hours per day adults use their strengths, the more likely they are to report having ample energy, feeling well-rested, being happy, smiling or laughing a lot, learning something interesting, and being treated with respect.[12]

These outcomes are universally desirable. Essentially, when we're playing to our strengths, things come more easily to us and feel natural, comfortable, and energizing. It's pretty clear to see how it would be helpful to know your strengths in everyday life, but even more so when you're facing adversity, a challenge, or a health crisis. Wouldn't you rather spend more time feeling energized and happy than stressed out and overwhelmed?

Mindset and Cancer

In addition to Gallup's body of work around strengths, I studied research related to cancer and mindset. Dr. Carol Dweck is a professor at Stanford University and most well-known for her influential book, *Mindset: The New Psychology of Success*.[13] She coined the term *growth mindset* and defined it as "the understanding that we can develop our abilities and intelligence." Her work has impacted millions in the worlds of education, business, and sports.

Compelling research has emerged from Stanford's Mind and Body Lab including a 2023 study, "Changing Cancer Mindsets: A Randomized Controlled Feasibility and Efficacy Trial."[14] The study had 361 participants

---

12 Susan Sorenson, Gallup (2014). "How Employees' Strengths Make Your Company Stronger." Available at: https://www.gallup.com/workplace/231605/employee-strengths-company-stronger.aspx.
13 Dweck, Carol S. (2006, 2016) *Mindset: The New Psychology of Success*. Random House.
14 Stanford University's Mind and Body Lab, "Changing Cancer Mindsets: A Randomized Controlled Feasibility and Efficacy Trial." Available at: https://mbl.stanford.edu/sites/g/files/sbiybj26571/files/media/file/psycho-oncology-2023-zion.pdf.

with newly diagnosed, nonmetastatic cancers from across the United States. Participants had a variety of cancers including breast, colon, prostate, lymphoma, leukemia, endometrial, lung, ovarian, pancreatic, thyroid, and melanoma. Half of the patients were randomly assigned to be in the Cancer Mindset Intervention (CMI) group. This group completed seven online training modules of about 2.5 total hours over 10 weeks. The modules targeted mindsets about cancer and the body, including short videos of cancer survivors sharing their experience and the importance of their mindset, and Stanford faculty shared the scientific framework of mindset. The modules also included reflective questions to help cancer patients turn their learnings into their own actionable strategies for their cancer experience. The other half of the patients were assigned to the Treatment as Usual (TAU) group and did not receive the training.

The researchers share that "Adopting the mindset that cancer is 'manageable' or even an 'opportunity to grow' may engender a sense of hope, meaning, and proactive engagement with treatment, while adopting the mindset that cancer is a 'catastrophe' may lead to despair and disengagement, making an already difficult time even more challenging." Without getting into the weeds of the data gathered, they found that the group who received the CMI training reported significant reductions in their endorsements of cancer-as-catastrophe and body-as-adversary mindsets and significant increases in their agreement with cancer-as-manageable, cancer-as-opportunity, body-as-capable, and body-as-responsive mindsets compared to the participants in the TAU group who did not receive the online training. The results from their study are powerful and concluded that "a brief intervention was effective at improving physical, social, emotional, and functional health–related quality of life, increasing adaptive coping behaviors, and reducing physical system distress in newly diagnosed cancer patients." Essentially, even when going through a cancer diagnosis and treatment, patients can learn how to improve their mindset, which in turn will improve their overall health and well-being.

To say I was excited when I discovered this CMI research is an understatement. I was familiar with Dr. Dweck and had read her famous book, but I had no idea this was being studied in the cancer arena. I was also encouraged to read a National Cancer Institute article, *Facing Forward: Life After Cancer Treatment.*[15]

> You might find that going through a crisis like cancer gives you renewed strength. "I feel good that I've found ways to cope," one colon cancer survivor said. "I also feel better able to handle any future problems that might come up. I have strength that I didn't know I had."

This cancer survivor's experience is an example of what researchers and psychologists call post-traumatic growth, which was pioneered by Dr. Lawrence Calhoun and Dr. Richard Tedeschi, professors of psychology at the University of North Carolina at Charlotte. Dr. Tedeschi said in his article "Growth after Trauma,"[16] "We've learned that negative experiences can spur positive change, including a recognition of personal strength, the exploration of new possibilities, improved relationships, a greater appreciation of life, and spiritual growth." He elaborated that post-traumatic growth is often seen in people who have endured war, bereavement, natural disasters, illnesses, and serious injuries. Additional research on post-traumatic growth in cancer survivors is being conducted around the world, and the findings will be beneficial to improve the cancer survivorship experience for the millions diagnosed annually.

Some of the most fascinating research-backed cancer material I've read since my diagnosis are the books *Radical Hope* and *Radical Remission*, by Kelly A. Turner, PhD.[17] Dr. Turner researched *Radical Remission* for her dissertation project and traveled to 10 countries, interviewing 20 radical remission survivors and 50 alternative healers. The *New York Times* bestselling author has now analyzed over 1,500 cases of radical

---

15 National Cancer Institute (March 2018). "Facing Forward: Life After Cancer Treatment." Available at: https://www.cancer.gov/publications/patient-education/facing-forward.

16 Tedeschi, Richard G. (July–August 2020) "Growth After Trauma," *Harvard Business Review*. Available at: https://hbr.org/2020/07/growth-after-trauma.

17 See Resources for Surviving Cancer with Your Strengths (page 335) for details of Kelly A. Turner's books.

remission, and her books are published in 23 countries. While her study focused on 75 factors that survivors identified as helping to defy their terminal cancer diagnosis, Dr. Turner focused on just nine or ten factors that were common to nearly all survivors. She shared, "These factors in the book include body, mind, and spirit interventions; the science behind the factor; a healing story from a survivor, and tips how cancer survivors can use the healing methods."[18] Her work received high praise from Dr. Keith Block, regarded as the father of integrative oncology, who commented on her work, "It provides a valuable service for cancer patients seeking foundational principles of self-care that will help them enhance their health and well-being both during and after physician-prescribed treatments."

Reading these fascinating examples of cancer and mindset research reassured me that we can take some control of our cancer experience through our actions and approach to mindset.

Your Cancer Experience, Your Mindset, and Your Strengths

Since receiving your cancer diagnosis, you may have experienced challenging feelings like overwhelm, anger, fear, worry, stress, anxiety, and depression. You are likely acquiring much new information, data, and thoughts, and are having to incorporate new appointments, behaviors, and routines into your life.

After reading this book, you will have an improved understanding of your strengths and how to leverage them during your cancer experience. You will read inspiring stories, ideas, and quotes from other cancer survivors on how they approached their cancer experience in a way that worked best for them, based on their strengths. You will have real actions to consider and feel more confident, stronger, resilient, and hopeful. Instead of being paralyzed with fear and worry, reading this will give

---

18 Radical Remission: https://www.radicalremission.com.

you an opportunity to do something about it. Playing to your strengths can help you navigate cancer with courage, dignity, and authenticity. It doesn't mean that it will be easy, or that you won't face challenges along the road, even when using your strengths. But you can still be engaged and energized when the path is difficult.

This book can serve as a compass, or an orienting tool for cancer-related ideas and advice. It offers you plenty of examples that, depending on your talents, may resonate with you. When you are driving someplace, you may enter an address into Google maps or another app on your phone. It gives you a variety of routes, and there is always one that is fastest. If navigating cancer authentically is our desired destination, then this book will provide you with the customized, most efficient route.

Remember playing the piñata game at birthday parties as a kid? You were blindfolded, spun around in circles a couple times, and given a stick to take a few swings at the piñata hanging from the ceiling or a tree. Some parents made it extra challenging by raising and lowering the piñata while the children's swing often got nothing but air. We all laughed, watching our friends clumsily swing and miss the festive piñata until the lucky winner finally made solid contact, the piñata broke, and we'd all rush to claim the candy and prizes covering the floor.

Receiving a cancer diagnosis can make you feel similarly disoriented and overwhelmed. There will be a ton of advice you could try but that might not feel like a solid hit for you. Rather than stumbling your way blindfolded and whacking away at gathering all the cancer advice and ideas, this book serves to remove the blindfold and, based on your strengths, turn you in the right direction as a starting point. It will help you feel a bit more grounded and regain your footing, when the Earth seems unsteady. We know your cancer experience can feel like a moving target, so orienting you toward your strengths will increase the likelihood you'll find ideas and advice that fit you. At a stressful and overwhelming time, this shortcut, so to speak, for considering helpful ways to adjust your mindset and take action during your cancer experience will save you time and energy when both are at a premium.

You are reading a book that will help you individually approach your cancer. This is because there is no one, right, way to navigate the disease. Just like cancer, we are complex, dynamic, and unique creatures. Capitalize on the beauty within you to make your cancer experience the smoothest, most efficient and fulfilling path possible. The pages that follow outline brief examples of how four cancer survivors have done just that. We are going to meet Holly, Dave, Mary Sue, and Tom. These survivors had various levels of strengths awareness: two had not taken the assessment, one was a longtime Gallup-Certified Strengths Coach, and one literally "wrote the book."

Holly

Holly's Top 5 Strengths:
Strategic—Competition—Achiever—Focus—Significance

Holly LaVallie was a vice president in marketing with a demanding leadership role, and a single mom raising two teenage daughters, when she received her breast cancer diagnosis. She shared, "As I was going through my diagnosis so many people said, 'Where are your emotions? Why are you being so pragmatic?' I started to wonder if maybe I was stuffing my emotions down. But when I took the CliftonStrengths assessment, it provided this incredible light for me. I realized, no, Holly, you are not stuffing things down. How you're handling the hardest thing you've been through is by leaning into your greatest strength, and you didn't even know that you were doing it. You're taking something extraordinarily complex and making it very simple, putting key milestones in place, and asking a lot of questions. The other part I learned from taking the assessment is that people with the Strategic strength go through all the potential outcomes, good and bad, and they weigh them out to find a range of risk, the highest upside and the lowest downside. When I very naturally did that with my diagnosis, I found out my risk is manageable. Now it's just a matter of managing it. I'm actually quite grateful because I thought I was stuffing some emotions. What you did by taking me through this strength assessment helped me recognize that I'm actually leaning on my greatest strength."

Holly beat cancer the way she lives her life—by asking questions, creating a plan, working hard, and demonstrating courage and perseverance while being an amazing mom and leader along the way.

Dave

Dave's Top 5 Strengths:
Achiever—Responsibility—Strategic—Includer—Activator

Dave Smith had been a friend of our family since the late nineties when his son Jason and Kent, now my husband, played basketball together at the University of Iowa. He was a man who stood out in a crowd not only because of his executive presence but also for how he made you feel welcome and part of the team. In the words of his family:

> Dave did not fit any molds, understandable, standing tall at six foot seven. He paved his own way and followed his own rules, one of which was "Better to ask for forgiveness than permission!" He had a commanding presence with the kindest demeanor, and a way of making everyone around him feel special, cared for, and loved.

So, when Dave received his Stage 4 pancreatic cancer diagnosis in June 2020, it left his family, colleagues, and wide circle of friends in confusion and disbelief. This disease and prognosis did not match the man on the receiving end.

When I shared the CliftonStrengths assessment with Dave in November 2020, he mentioned that his cancer diagnosis probably impacted his answers. But his son Jason and daughter-in-law Courtney felt the strengths were in line with how he lived his entire life—both before and during cancer. Jason shared, "*Loyal* was one of the most significant words to describe my dad. He built trust with his doctor immediately and told us, 'I trust Dr. C.' [Dr. Chandrikha Chandrasekharan]. She listened and gave me a lot of information. I felt very comfortable with her from the first meeting, so let's get started.'" Jason's description made it clear that Dave leveraged his Strategic and Activator strengths in evaluating the situation, factoring in all the complexities of the pandemic impacting cancer care, and not wasting any time in moving forward once he had built that trust with his doctor and care team. Jason acknowledged that if his dad had waited to start treatment or gone searching for a second opinion, the reality of facing cancer in 2020 may have led to even less time to treasure together as a family.

As Jason talked about how his dad managed his cancer diagnosis, treatment decisions, and advanced care planning he shared, "It's almost like he approached those last 11 months of his life similar to four quarters in a basketball game." As Jason effortlessly described each quarter and the type of activities and emotions involved, I felt like I was listening to a coach drawing up plays on a clipboard:

- 1st quarter: We were all shocked, stressed, and scrambling to figure out the prognosis and plan.
- 2nd quarter: Dad began easing into treatments. He and Mom were getting used to the process and understanding how his body was going to feel based on the impact of each treatment.
- 3rd quarter: This phase involved reflection and taking stock of "what all do I have to get done before my time is up?" Then Dad was checking all those things off the list.
- 4th quarter: Was all about "Let's do as many memorable things as possible and enjoy the time we have left while I'm feeling good." In fact, Dad even rented a party bus and took my mom, his daughter Jenny, myself, Courtney, and his four grandkids on the High Roller, the 550-foot giant Ferris wheel on the Las Vegas strip. After that, Dad and Mom renewed their wedding vows at the Little White Wedding Chapel in honor of their nearly 46 years together.

Dave's family shared many examples of his Achiever strength including how he wanted to do normal things during his treatment, such as playing golf with Barb and his father, visiting Las Vegas a few times, and working in his real estate development business until just over a month before he passed away in May 2021. In his career, Dave developed millions of square feet of real estate, primarily in the suburbs of Chicago and the Midwest, and was known for his honesty, integrity, and work ethic. When Jason and I wrapped up our conversation about his dad and how he was definitely living his strengths through his cancer experience, he reflected, "You know, we did some things for Dad like buying him a special shirt for infusions and getting those Big Dave black and gold bracelets for friends and family to wear. But I'm not sure we even asked him what he thought, of . . ." Jason's voice trailed off and he swallowed hard. "You're right. You almost have to do an assessment of what each person needs. It's not a track home-build . . . it's a custom development." Through the phone, I could tell Courtney was smiling when she reported that Dave really liked the bracelets. Kent added he was still inspired when he thought about Dave while wearing the bracelet on the golf course.

Big Dave beat cancer the way he lived life—by taking responsibility for decisions and plans, getting a lot done, surprising his grandkids with gifts, and making memories with the people he loved the most.

Mary Sue

Mary Sue's Top 5 Strengths:
Input—Connectedness—Ideation—Learner—Intellection

Mary Sue Ingraham is a breast cancer survivor, executive coach, and long-time Gallup-Certified Strengths Coach. When I spoke with her about how she effectively leveraged a variety of her strengths during her cancer experience, she shared, "There are different seasons of cancer. We may need different strengths at different times. There is not a one-size-fits-all approach. When you are reading and hearing everything about cancer, don't get ahead of yourself. You are an n of 1. I approached it like, 'This is my boat. I pick the people and supplies who join me.'" She continued:

> I recently heard Dr. Martin Seligman, a leading authority in the field of positive psychology, speak and he said, "Well-being is the purpose of life." This taught me that it's not selfish to tend to your own health and well-being. I also heard Harvard medical professor Dr. Alisha Moreland-Capuia speak at the Institute of

Coaching Conference. She encouraged us to "brush up against the edges of joy at least once daily," so I am incorporating more joy into my life.

Mary Sue beat cancer the way she lives her life—by gathering insights from experts, continually learning, spending time in nature, and focusing on joy and beautiful moments with her family.

Tom

Tom's Top 5 Strengths:
Futuristic—Significance—Strategic—Analytical—Focus

Tom Rath has written several international bestsellers; spent 13 years leading the strengths, employee engagement, and well-being work at Gallup; and is the grandson of Dr. Don Clifton. Together, they wrote *How Full Is Your Bucket?* just months before Don passed away. His book *StrengthsFinder 2.0* is Amazon's top-selling nonfiction book of all time. Other bestsellers include *Strengths Based Leadership, Are You Fully Charged?* and *Wellbeing: The Five Essential Elements.* Although Tom doesn't speak of this often, he is a cancer survivor and was diagnosed with Von Hippel-Lindau disease (VHL) at the age of 16. VHL typically runs in families, but his condition was a new mutation that affects just one in every 4,400,000 people and leads to rampant cancerous growth throughout the body. In his book *Eat Move Sleep*,[19] he shares the following powerful testimony about his approach to cancer:

> I have had annual exams and scans for over 20 years now and currently have small tumors in my kidneys, adrenal glands, pancreas, spine, and brain. Waiting around for active tumors to grow may sound nerve-racking. It could be, if I dwelled on the genetic condition that is beyond my control. Instead, I use these annual exams to stay focused on what I can do to decrease the

---

19 Rath, T., (2013) *Eat Move Sleep: How Small Choices Lead to Big Changes.* Missionday.

odds of my cancers growing and spreading. As each year goes by, I learn more about how I can eat, move, and sleep to improve my chances of living a long and healthy life. Then I apply what I learn to make better choices. I act as if my life depends on each decision. Because it does.

You can hear a few of Tom's strengths—such as Analytical, Focus, and Futuristic—coming through clearly in that message. Tom is beating cancer the way he lives his life—by analyzing research and data, connecting the daily decisions he makes to his future well-being, making significant contributions through his work, and prioritizing time with his family.

I've had the incredible opportunity to hear Tom deliver two keynote speeches in person. When he spoke at the Gallup Strengths Summit in July 2017, I sat in a crowd of 1200 people and listened attentively while tired and bald, with chemo racing through my body. I had just received my third of 16 rounds of chemo and had to be driven from Waterloo to Omaha to attend the conference because I was too tired to drive myself. Given my recent diagnosis and newfound appreciation for my mortality, it was so inspiring to hear him discuss the fragility of life and say, "We have today to use our time and talents." Out of character for me, I waited in line to talk with him after his keynote. I thanked him for his powerful message, mentioned I was in the midst of cancer treatment, and shared my idea for a book about using your strengths through cancer. When I asked him what he thought, he grinned slightly and said, "I like that idea. I'd like to see that."

Granted, I had no idea how to actually write a book or that it would take me over seven years to do so, but Tom's nod of validation gave me encouragement to stick with it. During that time, I continued to hear powerful stories of incredible cancer survivors like Holly, Dave, Mary Sue, and Tom. Just like them, you can use your strengths to improve your mindset, increase your confidence, and boost your energy levels during your cancer experience. You too can "beat" cancer in your own unique way.

How to Discover Your Strengths

This book is designed for you to pair with one or more of the options below so you can understand and use your strengths to get the most out of the book's personalized recommendations.

Choose one or more of these assessment options:
- **Take Gallup's CliftonStrengths assessment online.** Allow yourself 30 minutes of uninterrupted time to complete the assessment. This is the ideal option as it will be the fastest and most reliable, but it's not the only way to learn more about your strengths. The various assessment options are available on the Follow Your Strengths® Book page at https://www.followyourstrengths.com/book. You can purchase the Top 5 assessment for $24.99 or the Full 34 for $59.99. If you already have your Top 5 results and would like to see your full list of strengths, you can upgrade to the Full 34 for $49.99 and do not need to retake the assessment if you select that option. Additional products and assessments related to CliftonStrengths are located on the Follow Your Strengths® Resources page.

- **Retrieve previous CliftonStrengths assessment results if you have already taken the assessment.** It was referred to as the Strengths-Finder assessment beginning in 1999, for nearly 20 years, in case you remember it under its previous name. There is no need to retake the assessment unless that is your preference. If you'd like to access your prior results, go to https://www.gallup.com/cliftonstrengths and sign into your account. If you have any challenges, contact the Customer Support page at https://www.gallup.com/support.

- **Read the definitions of each of the 34 strengths and select around 10 that sound most like you.** You can also ask a few family members, coworkers, managers, or close friends to choose 10 that remind them of you. Look for overlap and trust your intuition.

As you learn the language of strengths, keep in mind that the same strength may look a little different between two people. For example, one cancer survivor may have Empathy and Harmony, whereas another may have Empathy and Competition. The way they display and express their Empathy strength is likely unique because of the other strengths that surround it. The intricacy of how your strengths influence one another is called theme dynamics. Essentially, we are all more than one thing, and the complexity of human talent is captured in the customized CliftonStrengths assessment reports. In fact, Gallup shares that "the odds of you and another person having the same 34 strengths in the same order is only one in 33 million!"[20]

If you choose to take the assessment, there are a variety of resources available on your online dashboard with your results. If you opt not to take the assessment, or want additional resources, consider completing one or more of the following exercises.

Five Clues to Talent

The framework Five Clues to Talent is in the incredible book, *Soar with Your Strengths,* coauthored by Paula Nelson and Dr. Donald Clifton, the inventor of the CliftonStrengths assessment and former Gallup CEO.

---

20 Asplund J., Gallup CliftonStrengths (November 5, 2021) "Uniquely You: How Your Strengths Set You Apart." Available at: https://www.gallup.com/cliftonstrengths/en/356810/strengths-set-apart.aspx.

They outline "five characteristics of a strength to help you scan your life for anything you have ever done well."

As you read the Five Clues below, don't restrict yourself to your current day-to-day life. Reflect on your childhood, school years, previous work experiences, and hobbies you've enjoyed throughout your life.

1. **Yearning:** Think of the activities you are pulled toward, like a magnetic attraction. Imagine how a golden retriever reaches for a tennis ball, runs after it, chases it down and eagerly drops it for the thrower to toss again. This is how yearnings may appear in our lives.
2. **Satisfaction:** What are some activities that you truly enjoy doing or have enjoyed previously in your lifetime?
3. **Rapid Learning:** What are some things or activities that you learned easily or completed easily but couldn't transfer that learning to others as easily?
4. **Glimpses of Excellence:** Consider everyday moments where you naturally shine. Where have people told you that you're great?
5. **Total Performance of Excellence:** Reflect on activities or experiences where you are in the zone and may even lose track of time. Dig deeper and get specific about what you're doing, where you're located, who else is involved, and the other characteristics that help to create this state of flow within you.

The Four E's

Gallup's CliftonStrengths framework outlines four signs that you are effectively utilizing your strengths: Ease, Excellence, Enjoyment, and Energy.

- **Ease:** The task or activity feels natural and effortless to you.
- **Excellence:** You perform at a high level.
- **Enjoyment:** You find pleasure in what you're doing.
- **Energy:** You feel energized rather than drained by the activity.

"These 4 E's," explained Gallup's *Called to Coach* podcast, "serve as a guide for individuals to recognize when they are operating within their 'strengths zone.'"[21] The concept is part of Gallup's broader strengths-based approach, which emphasizes focusing on and developing one's natural talents rather than trying to fix weaknesses. This philosophy suggests that when people lean into their strengths, they are more likely to experience these positive qualities of ease, excellence, enjoyment, and energy in their daily activities.

Study, Celebrate, and Relive Your Successes

In *Soar with Your Strengths*, the authors suggest three steps: visualize, write, and talk.

- **Picture it:** Visualize and mentally rehearse those activities that you feel are strengths.
- **Write about it:** Describe your strengths vividly by writing specifics about what you're doing, where you are located when this strength shines, what it feels like during and after this strength experience, and the type of feelings you have or feedback you're receiving that help you know this is a strength.
- **Talk about it:** Keep your strengths top of mind by talking about them to people you trust. Share what excites you about your strengths and brainstorm ways you can continue developing and improving these strengths.

---

21 Jessica Dawson, Gallup Called to Coach Webcast Series Season 8, Episode 9, "Lean Into the Right CliftonStrengths Theme at the Right Time." Available at: https://www.gallup.com/cliftonstrengths/en/287276/lean-right-cliftonstrengths-theme-right-time.aspx.

Book Structure

Each of the 34 CliftonStrengths chapters in Part Two includes *Gallup Definitions*, *Cancer Connections*, *Cancer Considerations*, and *Cancer Cautions* sections.

The *Gallup Definition* section that opens each chapter includes a short description, a long description, and a group of six to twelve characteristics of each strength. This content is Gallup's intellectual property and official terminology for each of the 34 CliftonStrengths.

The *Cancer Connections* section is an overview of how having a certain strength may impact you as a cancer survivor.

Cancer Considerations are ideas, recommendations, and reminders of actions you can take during your cancer experience. This includes stories and examples of how having this strength helped other cancer survivors feel energized, equipped, and empowered.

Cancer Cautions are things that could potentially challenge you during cancer, but they are not absolutes. This section serves as a heads-up, an early warning, and something to keep in mind as these challenges are things other cancer survivors have shared.

Part Three of the book is *Caregiver Considerations*. This section is based on the strengths of the cancer survivor, not the caregiver. It gives caregivers some insight into their loved one's perspective to reflect on, along with a few strengths-tailored questions to ask their loved one with cancer. And, of course, if a caregiver also wants to identify their own strengths, they should explore that too.

The connections, considerations, cautions, and examples in the book reflect various cancer phases, noted below. It's important to know these phases are rarely linear. In fact, you may repeat a few phases multiple times. If your diagnosis is Stage 4, you may continually receive some form of treatment, whether it's chemotherapy, medication, or proton therapy.

Here are a few high-level definitions or examples of experiences that may be included within each phase:

- **Testing:** biopsies, lab work, imaging.
- **Diagnosis:** staging of cancer, sharing the diagnosis, learning about treatment options.
- **Treatment:** chemotherapy, radiation, surgery, medication.
- **Recovery:** physical therapy, massage, exercise, post-surgery drain management.
- **Survivorship:** According to the National Cancer Institute, the government's primary funder of cancer research, this "focuses on the health and well-being of a person with cancer from the time of diagnosis until the end of life. This includes the physical, mental, emotional, social, and financial effects of cancer that begin at diagnosis and continue through treatment and beyond. The survivorship experience also includes issues related to follow-up care, late effects of treatment, cancer recurrence, second cancers, and quality of life. Family members, friends, and caregivers are also considered part of the survivorship experience."
- **Advocacy and volunteering:** mentoring a newly diagnosed cancer survivor, fundraising, participating in your local 5k cancer race, serving on the board of a cancer-related nonprofit, contacting state or federal political leaders, meeting with political leaders to share your concerns related to healthcare disparities.

How to Read this Book

Now that you have learned more about your strengths, begin by looking at those specific chapters. Notice:

- What ideas and recommendations feel easy and comfortable to you? Which ones will you try, and how will you monitor how things go?

- What feels uncomfortable or prickly to you? If these are in strengths chapters that are lower on your talent profile, or simply don't sound as much like you, you can always disregard the suggestion. If these are in the strengths chapters that are higher on your talent profile, or ones you thought sounded like you, that's okay too. Sometimes we have a hard time owning our strengths because in the past people have viewed them as weaknesses. You may have Communication as a strength but as a young person, a teacher may have complained that you talk too much. Explore why something feels uncomfortable and decide if it's worth digging into or discarding.
- If you're not sure about your strengths or are still gaining clarity, feel free to read all 34 strength chapters. You will see unique approaches and examples from other cancer survivors. Take note of the things that feel helpful and don't spend much time thinking about ideas that don't feel like a fit. I'd be surprised if you found all the recommendations equally helpful.

Additional Tips to Benefit from the Book

- **Set an intention:** Before you start reading, what is it you hope to gain? Write it down on a slip of paper. Use it as a bookmark or post it someplace you will see to remind you of your intention. Revisit it frequently, and don't feel obligated to do it all.
- **Take your time:** This book is intended to be a tool for you to reference and revisit over time. Feel free to skim, skip around, and make notes of your key insights along the way.
- **Revisit your strengths:** Review your strengths chapters in the book throughout the various phases of your cancer experience. A recommendation may resonate or fall flat with you depending on when you read it.
- **Avoid overwhelm:** You can take a bite-sized approach and read one strength each week or decide to read 10–15 pages at a time. If overwhelm begins to creep in, take a break.

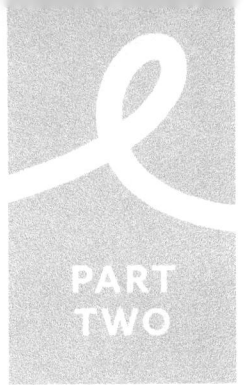

PART TWO

34 STRENGTHS, CANCER CONNECTIONS, CONSIDERATIONS, AND CAUTIONS

> I now understand that trying to be the next anyone is as foolish as it sounds. The shoes you dream of filling have already been worn ragged through their soles. You've got to step into your own kicks and do you.
>
> —*Alicia Keys, 15-time GRAMMY Award–winning artist and New York Times bestselling author of More Myself: A Journey*

Achiever

People exceptionally talented in the Achiever theme work hard and possess a great deal of stamina. They take immense satisfaction in being busy and productive.

Your Achiever theme helps explain your drive. You feel as if every day starts at zero. Every day, you must achieve something to feel good about yourself. And by "every day," you mean every single day—workdays, weekends, vacations. If a day passes without some form of achievement, no matter how small, you will feel frustrated and restless. You have a fire burning inside you. It pushes you to do more, to produce more. After each accomplishment, the fire dwindles for a moment, but it soon rekindles itself, pushing you toward the next accomplishment. Your relentless need for achievement might not be logical or even focused, but it will always be with you. You must learn to live with this whisper of discontent. It gives you the energy you need to work long hours without burning out. It is the jolt you can always count on to get started on new tasks and new challenges. It is the power

Many survivors do not feel like they're ever back to Life Before Cancer. The experience of having cancer changes you forever, and accepting that is also a strength.

supply you use to set the pace for yourself and others. Achiever is the theme that keeps you going.

Characteristics of Those with Achiever Talents

Driven	Intense	Productive
Independent	Diligent	Self-motivated
Ambitious		

Cancer Connection

You are likely somebody who works hard and gets a lot done. Cancer will test you in many ways. It may reduce the number of projects you can complete, your desire to do more, and the length of time you have energy to be productive. But it won't eliminate your intensity, passion, and drive. Given that there are many steps in a cancer treatment plan, you have a mental edge. Your natural state and where you feel best is when you're finishing tasks. This is absolutely a unique advantage because there are many opportunities to check things off during your cancer experience.

Globally, this is the most commonly occurring strength, with roughly 30% of people having this in their Top 5 results.[22] So, keep your eyes open for others like you who can appreciate your desire to keep working, stay busy, and get things done. They are the perfect people to provide active, productive support for you along the way, like driving you to your appointments, exercising with you, or bringing food by for dinner one night.

As a person who is driven to accomplish and has Achiever in my Top 10 strengths, I initially found it helpful to picture my treatment plan as phases to be completed. I have a hard time looking too far in advance,

---

22 Gallup CliftonStrengths, "Learn About the Science and Validity of CliftonStrengths." Available at: https://www.gallup.com/cliftonstrengths/en/253790/science-of-cliftonstrengths.aspx.

so keeping my focus on each phase helped me feel like I was hitting milestones and finishing something along the way. For example, I had four rounds of a very difficult chemotherapy called AC (Adriamycin and cyclophosphamide). As I progressed I would tell myself and others, "I'm 25% done," or "I'm halfway through this brutal part of chemo." As I think back on it, visualizing this as a separate phase was a way for me to measure progress and feel like I was accomplishing milestones along this tough stretch of the overarching cancer treatment plan.

Donna O'Brien, one of the first local breast cancer survivors who multiple friends introduced me to, was diagnosed at age 45 with invasive lobular breast cancer in 2008. Donna's treatment plan began with the removal of 26 lymph nodes, and she was informed that 21 of them were positive. She then had a single mastectomy, five months of chemotherapy, 35 radiation treatments, and a second mastectomy and reconstruction in 16 surgeries. She shared, "Given my Achiever talents, I have always been energized by checking things off my list. In fact, I made sure to get on the treadmill every single day during my treatment, even if it was just for five minutes. My son was playing college football during this time, and he coached me to picture my treatment plan as a football field and think of ways I was getting completions, first downs, touchdowns, and finishing each quarter of the game."

Because you're wired similarly to Donna and me, and have an innate need to feel productive, consider creating a visual representation of the cancer tasks in front of you. My sister made me a paper chain and numbered each link 1 through 16 to represent each round of chemotherapy. She urged me to crumple up each numbered link after that chemo session was finished, but they were too pretty for me to tear. Just the same, it was awesome to be able to track my progress along the chain, to see the light at the end of the tunnel, as I headed to my final few treatments. On the link for the final AC chemotherapy—it's referred to as the *Red Devil* by many women—my sister wrote the best message. "Adios, Red Devil!" Saying goodbye to a tough phase of your treatment process is an incredible feeling for people with this strength because we love to finish things and move on to what's next.

Cancer Considerations

Look for ways to work hard
As odd as this may sound, as you move through your healing plan, look for ways to work hard. Many people will be advising you to "slow down, take it easy, and *rest*." While *rest* generally isn't bad advice for cancer patients, it is not always the best advice for you because of your Achiever strength. This strength falls in the Executing domain, and what energizes you is completing tasks and getting things done. So don't hesitate to maintain that drive while you honor your healing needs.

Prioritize and be flexible
Prioritization is critical, perhaps more than ever before. Make sure the tasks you're planning to tackle truly belong on your list. Many cancer survivors still carry out their work as they go through treatment, whether by choice or necessity. If you are working, or continuing your typical day-to-day activities, consider adapting your schedule to better align with your stamina. When your treatment begins, it's helpful to keep a written record of your energy levels. Document when they drop, level out, and rise again. This knowledge will help you plan future activities accordingly.

I knew the first two days after chemotherapy would be relatively normal for me, but Days Four through Seven were rough. My energy levels were low, and I spent quite a bit of time in the recliner watching *This Is Us* episodes. That show got me through chemo because I had something to look forward to when I felt crummy. During my first type of chemotherapy, I'd get a burst of energy about eight to ten days after the infusion. I felt pretty good for the next four to six days until I went back for another round. Once I understood the typical patterns of my energy levels, I planned my work schedule around them. Being able to predict the good days, I knew I could run errands and meet up with friends for lunch or walks then.

Focus your attention

If you are taking time away from work or your typical day-to-day routines during treatment, this might be a good time to pay attention to what hasn't gotten much of your focus lately. Many people with Achiever talents report their relationships suffer when they pour so much time into working hard and accomplishing their goals. Perhaps this is a time to invest energy in relationships and areas of your life that haven't gotten as much of your time and focus. If you are working to a reduced schedule or from home more, what small home project have you been wanting to complete but never had the time? Cleaning out the coat closet may be just the project you need to get your mind off cancer and fuel your need for getting things done.

Create a cancer checklist

People with Achiever talents often make to-do lists and enjoy the thrill of checking things off their list. Would it be helpful for you to create a cancer checklist? As you endure key phases of your care, such as treatment steps and recovery, what goals do you want to keep your eye on to ensure completion? If you are fortunate to have a circle of support, put those people on your list. If you love checking things off your list, now is a great time to add things like *send thank you notes, call my sister,* or *go on a walk with my neighbor* to your list. You will love checking those things off your list, and your support team will love hearing from you and spending more time with you.

Build your team

Use your gift of working hard and getting things done to anticipate where you may need or like assistance along the way. More than ever, people are turning to you to understand what you see and how they can help make your visions a reality. They will be open to whatever you delegate in their direction. Is there somebody who can help you *hit send* or *close the book* on a project you've started? Engage them to help you finish what you can't do on your own right now. One survivor asked a close friend to take her fall decorations to storage and help her with putting winter decorations out around the house. She wanted to put more of her energy toward decorating the Christmas tree with her family. Our neighbor Sharon, an Achiever, endured a Stage 4 breast cancer diagnosis for 12 years. A team of her friends would gather in the yard early spring and late fall to do seasonal maintenance and keep her lawn and garden looking beautiful for her to enjoy. You will no doubt enjoy checking things off your list, but your friends will also get satisfaction from helping you by offering up a natural strength, their productivity.

Push a cause forward
Looking at the bigger picture, there is certainly a lot of work to be done in the cancer arena. You are wired to work hard. Is there something you could see yourself working on that could help with cancer awareness and prevention, research, or advocacy? For example, if you desire to influence legislation and policy, many steps must take place for meaningful change to be enacted. This reality is daunting and disheartening for many. However, your drive to complete a mission will help you continue pushing to move forward a cause or an issue related to cancer research or policy.

Cancer Cautions

Reassess your energy
Are your former productivity measures still realistic given your fatigue levels? As you plan your days and weeks, factor in your decreased energy. For example, if your typical Saturday used to involve working out at the gym, meeting a friend for coffee, shopping at the local farmer's market, and then getting groceries, is that still a reasonable expectation? I'm not saying, stop accomplishing tasks; however, consider shifting your thoughts about the amount of work you'll complete. Laura shared that she sometimes overdid things in an effort to make herself "feel normal" during her health crisis. Once she realized this, she intentionally practiced mindfulness to ensure she wasn't pushing herself too hard to the detriment of her health and recovery.

Partner with your supporters
Another great strategy is to get creative with your partnerships and support system. Are there ways where the work can still get done but you don't own 100% of the effort? Is there a project that somebody else could start and you finish? Or maybe there's something you'd prefer to start but need to outsource the finishing piece. What part of what project can be taken off your list? Ask your supporters to report back so you can all celebrate that task being done.

Explain your Achiever strength
Depending on your support system, people may worry you are pushing too hard or doing too much. It may help everyone if you explain that as ironic as it may sound, getting things done makes you feel better than staying idle. Inform your loved ones that what may exhaust other people actually gives you more energy.

Don't try to "finish cancer"
Given your love of to-do lists, you may have added a line item: Finish cancer. I apologize if this feels blunt to you, but cancer is going to be tough to completely check off your list. For most people, cancer is never finished. There is a spectrum of completion given the type and severity of your cancer, but it is important to note that this may not be something you ever consider *done*.

My treatment plan was mapped out from May through November, so I naïvely thought I just had to get through a tough six months. I even thought I was *done* after my surgery near Thanksgiving. I watched as my hair grew back, breathed a sigh of relief, and thought of my breast cancer as a scary event from the past. But the final part of my treatment included taking tamoxifen, a daily pill for five years. The side effects of that drug are fatigue, hot flashes, weight gain, and other menopausal symptoms even though I was only 40. While not debilitating, it still impacted my daily life for five years, nearly 2,000 days. I did not feel *done*.

Even if you have an early stage of cancer or a type that can effectively be removed via surgery, many survivors do not feel like they're ever back to Life Before Cancer, and that's okay. You will acquire many memories, stories, and possibly new friends along the way, and those will become an important part of your life. The experience of having cancer changes you forever, and accepting that is also a strength.

Activator

People exceptionally talented in the Activator theme can make things happen by turning thoughts into action. They want to do things now, rather than simply talk about them.

"When can we start?" This is a recurring question in your life. You are impatient for action. You understand that analysis has its uses and that debate and discussion can yield valuable insights. But deep down, you know that the only way to make things happen is to take action. Only action delivers results. Others may worry about unknown details or pending decisions, but this doesn't slow you down. You must take the next step. Once you make a decision, you can't help but do something. You learn by doing. You take action, you evaluate the outcome, and what you learn informs your next step. You know you will be judged not by what you say or think, but by what you do.

> I think everyone should be impatient about their health. Leveraging my Activator talents and advocating for myself saved my life.
>
> —*Carrie, kidney cancer survivor*

Characteristics of Those with Activator Talents

Impatient	Action-oriented	Catalytic
Fast	Influential	Initiating
Propulsive	Dynamic	

Cancer Connection

Chances are your patience will be greatly tested throughout this medical journey. As my Strengths teacher, Curt Liesveld, so eloquently described it, this is the "hate to wait" strength.[23] There is a lot of waiting involved in the medical process. It may look like any or many of the following:

- Waiting for your initial appointment
- Waiting for your pathology results
- Waiting for more information from your medical team
- Waiting to finalize your treatment plan
- Waiting to share the news with loved ones at the "right" time
- Waiting to get your blood drawn on chemo days
- Waiting to see if your lab results are good enough to receive chemo
- Waiting for your chemo "cocktail" to be mixed in the pharmacy
- Waiting for the chemo to hit you and waiting to see how you feel
- Waiting for clinical trials and medical advancements
- Waiting for your surgery date
- Waiting for the day cancer is behind you, if possible.

    People with Activator talents are often willing to make the first move while other survivors may be gathering more information or delaying the first treatment. While other patients may dread treatment, whether chemo, radiation, or surgery, your gut instinct is "Let's do this. Let's get

---

23 Gallup CliftonStrengths. "Activator: Learning to Love All 34 Talent Themes." Available at: https://www.gallup.com/cliftonstrengths/en/251432/activator-learning-love-talent-themes.aspx.

going." Don't take this talent for granted. You have a mental edge here, and this is absolutely a unique advantage for you as you move along your cancer experience.

Your Activator strength gives you an urgency to be naturally inclined to act and get started. You crave movement and feel best when you can get people or things moving through your influential presence and energy. There may have been times in your life where people referred to you as brave. You are likely more comfortable with risk than others. This natural inclination toward forward momentum will serve you well as you move through new medical experiences.

Activator is a Lesser Talent for me (number 32 of 34, to be clear). But I distinctly remember my impatience bubbling up the day after my diagnosis as I sat with a general surgeon for a second look at my results. I was thinking as I looked at him, "I have three tumors. You know how to operate. I'm free right now . . . or tonight . . . or during the middle of the night, for that matter! What do you say we just book an OR quick and take care of removing these bad boys?"

This isn't how it works, not even close. That meeting with the surgeon was on May 16. My double mastectomy surgery was November 16, exactly six months later, after 16 rounds of chemotherapy, dozens of doctor's appointments, and hours of waiting. I can only imagine my close friends with the Activator strength. They'd have pressed a scalpel into that surgeon's hands, urging, "Let's go!"

Michelle, a breast cancer survivor with Activator talents, shared with me, "The longer I had to wait to tell my kids about my breast cancer diagnosis, the harder it was for me. Although I hated waiting to share the news, I simply didn't want to tell them until we had a plan. The entire experience brought home the fact that you just don't know when your last day will be. Life is too short, so I took the approach of making memories now because that is what's most important."

In fact, Michelle went to Disney World with her kids while enduring treatment. While she initially waited to share the news with them, she was able to dial up that Activator strength by sharing experiences and making memories. She didn't let her cancer diagnosis cause her to wait on anything!

Carrie, a kidney cancer survivor, told me, "Strengths can be a language for people to advocate for themselves. The definition of Activator used to include the word *impatience*. I suddenly had an appreciation for my impatience. I had that appreciation for my ability to influence, to go back to that doctor, and to do my own research. I was able to use my voice and my talents to advocate for myself and my health. Whether you have Activator talents or not, I think everyone should be impatient about their health. Our companies aren't going to do it for us, the healthcare system is not set up to do it for us, and our government will not do it for us. We have access to information. I was proud of myself. I just asked the questions and luckily had a doctor who was willing to go there with me and we found it."

Thanks to her pushing for further testing for her gastrointestinal pain, Carrie's kidney cancer was luckily discovered at Stage 1. A scan revealed the tumor, which was separate from her initial concerns. "Ultimately, leveraging my Activator talents and advocating for myself saved my life."

Cancer Considerations

Get started

You'll be receiving a lot of advice from medical professionals and possibly even more from family, friends, and other sources. Your gift is *starting*. Try out an idea. Maybe it's beginning a walking routine, meditation, a change in your diet, or adding a spiritual practice. Whereas many people may be overwhelmed by all the advice pouring in, you will jump in. You are often the one encouraging others, "What will it hurt?" Give yoga or a local support group a try. You don't have to do it forever. If something new sticks and helps you feel stronger, implement a plan or structure for your new activity to become a habit. Trust your natural talent for starting in this new strange territory.

Focus on fresh starts

You may want to see each phase of treatment as a new beginning rather than as one long block of time. It's an intentional mental shift to see chemo, surgery, radiation, recovery—whatever you may be doing to heal—as something new. This may give you energy to purposely think of each phase as something fresh to start. It may not be as sexy as starting a business, a church, a project, or a new social group but it will tap into your natural Activator strength.

Invigorate your supporters

You are naturally aware of fresh opportunities and have the gift of creating energy for others to act and influencing them to get going. Now, more than ever, people are turning to you to understand where to start, and they will be open to whatever you delegate their direction. What home or family project would you like somebody to start or help you start, like addressing and mailing your holiday cards, or meal prepping healthy foods for the week? Is there anything you already started, at work or home, that you need to pass the baton to somebody else to finish? Does your cancer diagnosis present any new possibilities? Are there any cancer-related programs, products, nonprofits, or legislation you wish were in place but currently do not exist? Perhaps you want nothing to do with the cancer arena, but this life-altering event has shined a brighter light on other passion projects. Can you leverage your contagious energy to get the ball rolling on any of these initiatives?

Cancer Cautions

Consider your options

Given your innate preference for action and learning by doing, you may need to slow down to carefully consider the treatment options presented. Enlist a supporter to help you weigh your alternatives and potentially obtain a second opinion. Most people want to move forward quickly when initially diagnosed with cancer, and this inclination is heightened in those with the Activator strength. Challenge yourself to consider your options, alternatives, and consequences of your decisions before committing to a specific healthcare organization, physician, or treatment plan. This recommendation is not in any way suggesting you delay important medical treatment. It is a reminder to leverage all your resources while evaluating the best treatment plan for you. Then go!

Evaluate your resources and reprioritize

Be strategic regarding what needs to be started now and if you have the energy to do it or need to enlist support. Your Activator strength typically brings a lot of energy to others, but this may be compromised by cancer. For example, if you typically initiate five home projects every weekend, either dial your expectations back to starting three or enlist the help of a friend or family member to help with the remaining two projects. The recommendation is not to hit pause on everything until you complete your treatment. It's to evaluate if there is anything you can delay or take off your list.

Explain your Activator strength

Your gift is in starting and acting with a sense of urgency and often inspiring others in the process. Keep in mind that those close to you, potentially including family members, friends, and colleagues, may take longer to process your diagnosis than you do. Whereas you may be in a hurry to get started with treatment, it may take your support team time to catch up to you. Do your best to communicate to your team of supporters your thought process and desire to move forward.

Adaptability

People exceptionally talented in the Adaptability theme prefer to go with the flow. They take things as they come and discover the future one day at a time.

You live in the moment. You don't see the future as a fixed destination. Instead, you see it as a place that you create out of the choices you make right now, one decision at a time. This doesn't mean you don't have plans. But because of your strong Adaptability, you respond willingly to the demands of the moment even if they pull you away from your plans. You are naturally composed and levelheaded, and you rarely get flustered. You don't resent sudden requests or unforeseen detours. You expect them. On some level, you look forward to them. Your ability to navigate change and respond quickly to uncertainty while remaining calm reassures others and builds confidence and stability during times of transition or confusion. You are, at heart, a flexible, unflappable person who can stay productive when the demands of work and life are pulling you in many different directions at once.

If I could have chosen my top strengths on the day of my diagnosis, Adaptability would have been a first-round pick for me. There is beauty in living each day as it unfolds and realizing that all we are promised is today.

—Traci McCausland

Characteristics of Those with Adaptability Talents

Flexible	Easygoing	In the moment
Agreeable	Responsive	Present
Spontaneous	Existential	

Cancer Connection

You have the gift of remaining calm in the midst of chaos, in addition to responding and moving forward when faced with surprises. You are great at reacting to change and living in the moment. Your gift will be incredibly helpful for you while dealing with your cancer diagnosis as even the smoothest-laid treatment plans will likely involve a few twists and turns. This natural ability of yours to be flexible will impress, amaze, and inspire those around you. In fact, the strength of Adaptability falls in the Relationship Building domain. Your circle will be looking for ways they can help you while simultaneously learning from your example the entire way.

Shortly after my cancer diagnosis, I challenged myself to leverage my strengths to improve my mindset and energy levels. I gave quite a bit of thought to all 34 strengths, not just those high on my list. Adaptability consistently made its way to the top of the wish list. If I could have chosen my top strengths on the day of my diagnosis, Adaptability would have been a first-round pick for me. There is beauty in living each day as it unfolds and realizing that all we are promised is today.

A cancer diagnosis creates a sense of urgency to make decisions about your health and healing. You are a natural at responding to urgent situations and better equipped to handle this pressure than others who are less adaptable. Most of us are not flexible and not huge fans of change, but you are an exception to the rule. Although receiving a cancer diagnosis can feel incredibly crummy, your strength of Adaptability makes you a winner in the strengths lottery. You have an edge because of your ability to handle chaos and be open to change. This is so valuable for you because not only will you be experiencing a lot of change related to your health and body, but you will have to make some shifts in your daily life as well.

Cancer Considerations

You are good with rapid change

The healthcare system runs on appointments, and not always on time. You've been thrust into a whirlwind of activity including making appointments, sitting in waiting rooms, meeting with your care team, receiving treatment, picking up prescriptions, and probably rescheduling appointments for reasons often outside your control. This new workload is a lot for anyone to manage and is especially difficult for individuals who are used to being in control of their schedules. Given your natural inclination to be responsive and flexible, you have the power to handle these schedule shifts and changes remarkably.

One breast cancer survivor, Melanie, opted to delay her treatment slightly to move from a local provider to Mayo Clinic in Minnesota for treatment. She had an extensive family history of cancer and lost her grandma, aunt, and mom to the disease. Given the advanced level of expertise at Mayo Clinic, Melanie feels like she made a good decision by listening to her instinct to delay her local treatment option, be flexible, and pursue care out of town at Mayo. She got into a rhythm of understanding her daily energy levels and figured out when she could do things and when she couldn't. She called the days she didn't feel good her "down days," and said they were initially on the weekends, thankfully, but crept into Fridays the longer her treatment progressed. Once, she had gallstone pancreatitis. She needed to have her gallbladder removed, and that pushed one of her chemo infusions out. Although a little annoyed by this extra health issue, Mel calmly stated, "I feel like I have been going with the flow because that's all you can do, I guess."

If you read books and articles discussing your disease, you will often see it referred to as a "cancer journey," "cancer battle," or a "walk through cancer." The path is rarely linear for a patient and no two experiences are identical. Upon receiving a cancer diagnosis, most patients are given their cancer treatment plan. For example, your plan may include chemotherapy, surgery, and radiation in that order. Another patient's plan may involve surgery before chemotherapy. And a third patient may not do chemotherapy but will do surgery followed by radiation. Your care team will outline your care plan and timeline. Have you ever heard the phrase, "Plans are made to be broken?" Keep this expression in mind as you face changes along your treatment path. Patients may experience schedule shifts, medication updates, long wait times, and even physician changes. None of these were part of the original roadmap, but you will shine as you maneuver your way through these revisions like a pro.

There will also be many adjustments to your life outside of your medical schedule. For example, you may need to adjust your work schedule and daily routines because you don't feel well or have enough energy. You may have had commitments, goals, or even vacation plans that need to be revised. Some cancer patients are faced with difficult decision-making regarding fertility and family planning. Your appearance may also change. Depending on the type of cancer you're dealing with, this could include hair loss, skin changes, scars, or loss of a body part. Leverage your Adaptability talents to manage these twists and turns along your own cancer path.

Add routine if it helps your health

You are good with NOW, and may not typically look ahead to six months, one year, or five years down the road. Who can help you look toward the future with hope if you're consumed with the unpleasantness of the present? Is there an area in your life where you would like to have a more structured daily or weekly plan? Even though you are used to living life with a flexible plan, adding a bit more routine in your life could feel comforting. For example, if you want to incorporate more exercise into your life, do you need help creating a walking or strength training schedule? Do you have a colleague or friend who would love to help you design this plan? As you may not need to be told, this plan is not set in stone and can shift however you see fit. If a more spontaneous activity with others, like a pickup pickleball game or a quick round of golf, motivates you more than a plan, add those experiences into your life as well. Don't let the fear of rigidity stop you from making plans that will improve your health and well-being.

Adopt new products or activities
The advancements in modern medicine are incredible. There are new drugs, therapies, processes, policies, and organizations being created or improved daily. Given your natural inclination to be an early adopter, is there anything new or cutting-edge that could improve your condition? I've had many friends participate in clinical trials or try new cancer-related products. One example is Cooling Caps, devices that cool your scalp and reduce the amount of chemotherapy that reaches your follicles.[24] This, in turn, reduces hair loss and helps cancer survivors keep some or most of their hair during chemo.

What could you bring into your life, on the medical or even personal front, that may energize you and improve your current state? Challenge yourself to think of unique steps or activities that will aid in your healing.

Cancer Cautions

Communicate your one-day-at-a-time mindset
Your gift is in responding to change and living in the moment. It will be incredibly helpful for you while dealing with cancer. Although friends and family see you as flexible and laid back, keep in mind that they may not possess a similar temperament. Those close to you, including family members, friends, and colleagues, may take longer to process and accept this diagnosis and treatment plan than you do. Do your best to communicate your thought process and one-day-at-a-time mindset to your team of supporters. Be prepared to be patient for them to catch up to you, but the timeline is yours to own. Move forward whenever you are ready.

---

24 American Cancer Society, "Cold Caps and Scalp Cooling." Available at: https://www.cancer.org/cancer/managing-cancer/side-effects/hair-skin-nails/hair-loss/cold-caps.html.

Seek resources for forward-planning

Receiving the news of a cancer diagnosis is one of the toughest challenges people face in their lives. The news can be shocking, sad, and stressful. While your Adaptability strength will be much more of a help than a hindrance to you, make a conscious mental note that you are walking through one of the hardest times in your life. It can be daunting and overwhelming to be a cancer patient, so imagine the moments beyond receiving this news and enduring the difficult treatments. Your strength lies in dealing with the present, but remind yourself not to get stuck in it. You probably have some decisions and plans to make around future events.

For example, your surgery may not be scheduled for five months, but you may need to anticipate and plan how that procedure, recovery, and potential side effects will impact your day-to-day life. You may need to purchase supplies, take time away from work, ask somebody to drive you to follow-up appointments, or find a person to help with your post-surgical care and medication management. These are not activities that you can figure out on the fly or just wing it when those days arrive. Checklists, ideally with timelines included, will be especially helpful for you during these stressful times. If planning that far in advance is too difficult for you, reach out to your caregiver or support team for resources and advice on how to start and move forward.

Advocate for your needs

As with any medical condition, it is important to be your own advocate for your health. You may not be used to driving change, speaking up, or challenging authority. Now is a critical time to sit in the driver's seat or invite a member of your support system to take the wheel. Examples of taking the initiative with your care team include preparing questions before your appointment, sharing any frustrations, clarifying next steps, or initiating a schedule change.

Analytical

People exceptionally talented in the Analytical theme search for reasons and causes. They have the ability to think about all of the factors that might affect a situation.

Your Analytical theme challenges other people: "Prove it. Show me why what you are claiming is true." You are a logical, objective, and rigorous thinker. You trust data, numbers, and facts because they have no agenda. Your mind understands them. So using data, you search for connections. You want to understand how certain patterns affect one another and how all the variables work together. Always looking for the truth, you peel the layers back until gradually, you reveal the root cause or causes. Others depend on your rigorous thinking to evaluate their ideas. With strong Analytical, you can be skeptical, and you will not be convinced until you see solid proof.

Your Analytical strength will help you distill the information into what you most need to know and use right now. Stay tapped into this critical and objective approach, as you have many important decisions ahead.

Characteristics of Those with Analytical Talents

Objective	Data-driven	Skeptical
Scientific	Numbers-oriented	Dispassionate
Questioning		

Cancer Connection

A cancer diagnosis can stir up a spectrum of emotions in a person, from shock, fear, sadness, and anger to hope, gratitude, and optimism. People with Analytical as a strength tend to rely on what's known, true, accurate, and proven. *Emotional* is typically not a word used to describe people with this strength. In contrast, you are seen as objective, logical, and may even distance yourself from emotions to rely instead on data and facts.

While those around you may be swirling in all kinds of feelings and emotions because of your diagnosis, you may feel calm, thoughtful, and steady. When faced with adversity or difficult setbacks, you zoom out and examine the big picture, uncover what caused the problem, and evaluate your options to move forward. You take an objective, fact-based approach to problems and will feel best when addressing your cancer diagnosis and treatment options in this manner. Traci, a cancer survivor shared, "I try to go into my appointments with no expectations or predictions. For me, filling my head with too many scenarios is not productive or helpful." She explained how she takes a serious and intentional approach to sorting through cancer information and does her best to filter out anything not related to the topic she is searching. Traci shared that during one of her searches, "I found a site that talked about recurrence data and statistics. It caught me off guard at first, and then I reminded myself, 'Yeah, okay. I'm not looking for that data now. I'll stick that in my back pocket for later.'"

You were probably the kid growing up who delighted, and—let's be real—sometimes fatigued your teachers and family members with questions like "Why? How do you know?" The Analytical strength falls

Analytical

in the Strategic Thinking domain, and this inquisitive approach to life has probably helped you make some well-informed decisions. There's no doubt this curious mind of yours will work to your advantage as you navigate your cancer experience.

One question from cancer survivors that has surprised me is "Why not me?" This strikes me as the kind of response someone with the Analytical strength might have. Katie Couric, an award-winning American journalist and co-founder of Stand Up to Cancer has made it her mission to share the latest cancer data, statistics, research, and recommendations. She announced her breast cancer diagnosis in an article titled "Why NOT Me?"[25] I have no idea if Analytical is high on Katie Couric's list of strengths, but I do know that her journalistic approach to talking about the disease has helped thousands of people. She is no stranger to cancer. Her sister died from pancreatic cancer; her mother-in-law from ovarian cancer; her mother had mantle cell non-Hodgkin lymphoma; and her father, prostate cancer. Heartbreakingly, Couric's first husband and father of her two daughters, Jay Monahan, passed away from colon cancer in 1998 at 41. A few years later, Katie underwent a colonoscopy live on *The TODAY Show* and called herself the "Screen Queen." Although that nickname is funny, her courageous decision to be that vulnerable undoubtedly saved lives as the number of colonoscopies increased by 20% after her segment.

It was this familiarity with cancer that "quickly shifted her mood from disbelief to resignation" when she got her own diagnosis. "Given my family's history of cancer, why should I be spared? My reaction went from *Why me?* to *Why not me?*"

As most cancer survivors know, the day you are diagnosed is a day where information comes at you fast and furious. You will receive information from medical professionals, friends, and family, and some you will likely acquire on your own. Your Analytical strength will help you distill the information into what you most need to know and use right

---

25 Couric, K., Kate Couric Media, "Why NOT Me?" (2022). Available at: https://katiecouric.com/news/katie-couric-has-breast-cancer/.

now. You will have a strong sense of what information is helpful and what is distracting. Stay tapped into this critical and objective approach as you have many important decisions ahead. Do your part in asking the right questions, allowing yourself time to think, and reaching out for help when you need it.

Cancer Considerations

Ask questions; require good answers
According to the Gallup Organization, "before taking action, you ask the right questions of the right people." Navigating your cancer diagnosis will present you with numerous opportunities to utilize this skillset. Depending on the cancer institution, you may have limited time to meet with your oncologist and other members of your care team. Be ready with excellent questions. Push whomever you interact with to deliver satisfying answers.

Catherine, a Canadian Gallup-Certified Strengths Coach and cancer survivor with Analytical as a strength, shared:

> I actively participated with my care team and came prepared to ask questions. This helped me feel that I had control over my health and my fate. This was, seemingly ironically, a very empowering time for me. Using my Analytical strength made the experience a lot less scary because I received the knowledge that engendered the confidence that I needed to proceed through the journey.

Create an information collection plan
You thrive on data, logic, and credible sources of information in all aspects of your life. Facing a cancer diagnosis will be no different. Given the vast amount of information on the topic of cancer online, be critical about which sources you consume to ensure the input is accurate. Develop a plan for analyzing all the information and resources you will

receive. Create a system where you can collect the websites, books, or articles that are most helpful to you. In some cases, decisions need to be made quickly, so be prepared to allow yourself enough time and space to do your best thinking.

Simplify the complex
Receiving a cancer diagnosis, examining treatment options, and moving forward with a plan presents you with a lot of decisions to navigate. It feels very dynamic with many moving pieces and can be overwhelming. This leads many cancer survivors to feel confused, and some even hesitate to move forward with their care. You have the gift of simplifying the complex and reducing a large amount of information to the more digestible key points. Your tremendous ability to critically examine various medical scenarios and treatment options is valuable, allowing you to make decisions and gain forward momentum. Your objective approach to life will set you up to navigate these emotions better than most. Embrace this gift.

Share your Analytical strength
Share with your medical care team that you are analytical. Likely some of your doctors and caregivers share this strength. Explain that you are not intimidated by facts and data; in fact, you thrive on them and welcome them into your care discussions. Your logical approach to medical decisions will be refreshing for your care team. They will enjoy your inquisitive nature and the exchange of facts, knowledge, and insights about your care.

Use your critical thinking
Cancer is a complex and unique disease with over 100 different types. You will likely hear advice, stories, and insight from friends and family as everyone has been touched by cancer in one form or another. Some will be applicable, and others will be irrelevant. People are trying their best to be helpful to you, and your ability to critically examine information will serve you well as you analyze what helps and what you can ignore.

Dig in on the research and data

Where are you dissatisfied with the cancer data, statistics, and outcomes? Is this an arena where you want to take a deeper dive or are you willing to let it go? There may be causes or organizations you're drawn to that are working to answer difficult questions related to cancer treatment. For example, you may have a rare cancer and question the lack of resources dedicated to it, or you may uncover health disparity data and want to help the underserved. One sign of a talent is when you continually return to a topic or activity. If you find yourself unable to let go of certain issues or alarming data points, that may be a clue for you to put your Analytical strength to use and do some investigating. It may or may not be something you stick with, but the process of uncovering more details and insights will fill your bucket regardless.

Cancer Cautions

Be prepared for ambiguity

You are exceptional at searching for cause and effect for events and situations. While this is one of your greatest gifts, you need to manage this tendency during cancer. For many cancer patients, the cause of their disease is unknown or speculative. You may face side effects from your treatment where the cause cannot be definitively traced. Be prepared to face ambiguity along the way.

You love proof. During your cancer journey, you may be confronted with decisions where proof does not currently exist. Push your medical team to provide you with the best data available now and coach yourself by gathering the latest research while letting go of that desire for exactness in a situation where it doesn't exist. You feel that knowledge is power and are not a fan of guesswork. You are more of an exacting type than a "close enough" type. Be prepared that your desire for exactness may not always be honored as you learn data, estimates, and percentages. Remind yourself there are many unanswered questions related to cancer, and you may have to move forward with care decisions without all the answers.

Beware of paralysis by analysis

As you are confronted with countless scenarios to consider and decisions to be made, be aware of your tendency to gather more information before making decisions. While this is one of your top strengths, beware of overthinking, overanalyzing, and the dreaded paralysis by analysis. Set deadlines for your decisions or partner with somebody who can help you move forward. Be careful not to delay critical treatment if you find yourself overwhelmed by analyzing information.

Explain your Analytical strength

Your loved ones and support system may be more emotional about your diagnosis and difficult treatment side effects than you. In fact, they may be confused at how steady and perhaps neutral you are as you process your healthcare situation. It would be helpful for them to hear more from you about how this calm and objective style of yours is one of your strengths. Explain that although you may have feelings of sadness, fear, and anxiety, you are at your best when you can take a logical, objective, and even dispassionate approach to thinking through situations. Reassure them you aren't in denial but instead have a natural preference for logic and facts.

Arranger

People exceptionally talented in the Arranger theme are both organized and flexible. They enjoy figuring out how to align people and resources to get the best results.

Cancer has a way of piling on to your to-do list with appointments, phone calls to make, and resources to read. Your Arranger strength thrives in complex situations, and you will naturally find the perfect configuration for the people and processes involved in your cancer experience.

You are a conductor. When faced with a complex situation involving many variables, you enjoy managing them all—aligning and realigning them until you are sure you have found the most productive configuration possible. In your mind, there is nothing special about what you are doing. You are simply trying to figure out the best way to get things done. Whether you are changing travel schedules at the last minute because of a better fare or considering just the right combination of people and resources to accomplish a new project, you are a shining example of effective flexibility. When confronted with the unexpected, some complain that plans cannot be changed, while others find comfort in existing rules or procedures. You don't do either. Instead, you jump into the confusion, devise new options, look for new paths of least resistance, and figure out new partnerships—because after all, there might just be a better way.

Characteristics of Those with Arranger Talents

Flexible	Controlling	Multi-thinking
Real time	Interactive	Collaborative
Configuring	Resourceful	

Cancer Connection

Your treatment plan will present many opportunities for you to leverage your Arranger talents. There are a lot of moving pieces including learning more about your diagnosis and evaluating your medical options while managing your daily responsibilities. You naturally shift gears, adapt, and change to work toward productivity and the best outcomes. You are gifted in initiating change. Respect that gift and embrace it for the best possible plan—at least for now, until things change again. Keep in mind that the complexity of managing a cancer diagnosis and evolving a treatment plan is where your natural talents will work in your favor.

You can take the lead in directing small things that create efficiency for your health. For example, I asked my husband and friends who drove me to chemo appointments to drop me at the front door of the hospital while they parked the car and carried in bags or heavier items. This is a simple example, but it got me to my appointments quicker and gave them something to do other than sitting longer in a waiting room. Win-win!

Toward the end of my 16-round chemotherapy regimen, my fatigue had mounted. I continued to work part-time and deliver training workshops across the state. On three occasions, I enlisted help from my mom to drive. One trip I was exhausted and slept the entire time and on another, I reviewed my presentation. Mom and I both have the Arranger strength, and we smile as we affectionately referred to those experiences as "Driving Miss Traci."

My good friend, Liz, also shares the strength of Arranger. She was eager to help me coordinate something and offered to line up drivers for my chemo treatments. I knew I could manage that task myself, but I mentioned to her I could use some help writing thank-you cards. Before I knew it, Liz coordinated an evening where four girlfriends came to the house, we ate sushi, and knocked out a bunch of thank-you notes together. The night gave me so much energy because we got a lot done and did it efficiently, together.

One cancer survivor, Michelle, has the strength of Arranger and she had her friends and family join her for a cancer fundraising walk. She registered the team and ordered customized shirts for her squad. I organized a Farewell to Hair party where 30 women joined me at the salon and Sadika cut my hair short the week before chemotherapy took it all. I also hosted a party between my 15th and 16th chemo at our house for about 75 people after the local Beyond Pink TEAM Annual Pink Ribbon Run. The party was a great celebration after the 5k, complete with waffle makers and a donut wall. It was a blast to coordinate, and some great friends helped pull it all together.

These two events were two of my favorite days during my months of treatment. Most books for cancer survivors don't suggest hosting your own parties, and people assume that would be a burden and stressful. But Michelle and I had both played the role of social coordinator with our families and friends over the years, so we figured "Why stop now?" These activities were fairly easy for us to manage, kept us productive during our treatment phase, and were great ways to bring our supporters together.

Cancer Considerations

You thrive in complexity

You are great at managing multiple tasks, priorities, and responsibilities. Cancer has a way of piling on to your to-do list with appointments, phone calls to make, and resources to read. The sheer volume of new information and tasks that are launched your way upon receiving a cancer diagnosis are overwhelming to most. Many individuals are overcome with fear, fatigue, and paralysis by analysis when facing a cancer diagnosis. Keep in mind that your Arranger strength thrives in complex situations, and you will naturally find the perfect configuration for the people and processes involved in your cancer experience.

Curt Liesveld, my Strengths teacher at Gallup, explained that for people with Arranger talents "More is often better."[26] While some may prefer to solely focus on their cancer treatment plan, you may thrive with more activities and projects to go along with your medical appointments. I know multiple cancer survivors with Arranger strengths who continued working, attending their children's events, and serving on local committees. As your energy allows, keep what you can spinning on your plates. Many may dissuade you from participating, but you know yourself best and more, may in fact, be better for you.

Acknowledge your flexibility

Your treatment plan and regularity of appointments could quickly feel stale and boring to you as you thrive in dynamic environments. But you will likely hit a day when your chemo or other treatment is delayed, and you have to wait longer than usual. This change in routine would fluster and frustrate many, but you can effortlessly adapt your expectations because you're used to naturally shifting gears. Embrace this flexibility of yours and give yourself a mental high five as you easily navigate changes in days, times, medicines, and treatments. The very thing that will drain many survivors will barely register as a bump in the road for you.

Your thoughts and mindset will naturally shift over the weeks and months after receiving your diagnosis and starting treatment. Keep in mind that your plans will, and arguably, should change as you adapt

---

[26] Gallup CliftonStrengths. "Arranger: Learning to Love All 34 Talent Themes." Available at: https://www.gallup.com/cliftonstrengths/en/251312/arranger-learning-love-talent-themes.aspx.

and learn more along the way. Your initial course of action may change once you begin chemo, have surgery, or start radiation. You are naturally courageous in times of change. Honor your talent of evaluating the current state and making seamless changes. Consider this your building-the-plane-while-flying-it moment.

Monitor what works and build your plan
After you get a feel for your treatment days, devise the best schedule to optimize your health. If you notice that you do best when completing certain tasks or being around certain people, try to duplicate those efforts on future treatment days. Pay attention to when it is best for you to eat, exercise, reflect, nap, or sleep. When do you have the best energy levels during and after those activities? For example, do you like to take a walk first thing in the morning before you begin your day? Or do you prefer an evening walk after dinner has settled and the kitchen is cleaned? If there is a clear winner for your preferred time of day, build your days around that plan and invite friends, family members, podcasts, or solitude to join you on your walk. Look for the patterns and devise plans and systems that create the best schedule and feelings for you. This is good advice for all cancer survivors, but it's an especially important reminder for you with your Arranger strength because you are always looking for ways to optimize your schedule and add efficiency to your life.

Cancer Cautions

Can you take off a hat, or two?
You probably wear a lot of different hats. Many people with the strength of Arranger often hear "How do you do so much?" While you are navigating your cancer diagnosis and treatment plan, do you need to continue wearing *all* your hats? Are there any roles you can let go of or reduce your time commitment to during this time in your life?

Mix it up to avoid boredom

You thrive during times of change and will probably get bored during portions of your treatment plan that feel too predictable or repetitive. Find ways to make the same thing feel new. For example, you may have 12 weeks of the same kind of chemo treatment. How could you bring some variation into these to avoid feeling the dread of sameness? Could you bring different people with you? Could you plan different activities to go along with those days, such as reading one day and watching a TV show another? Like a DJ spinning records, find ways to mix it up and make the same experiences feel brand-new.

Explain your Arranger strength

Your natural preference may be to stay busy. You may get energized by having a lot to do and a tight timeline for completion. This may appear like overdoing it to your loved ones, and they will encourage you to take it easy or not take on so much. Be prepared to explain to them that being busy and efficient makes you feel good. They'll care about how you're feeling, so don't hesitate to explain that being busy is better for you, counterintuitively.

You are flexible and nimble and will likely move into the chaos that is cancer quicker than most. Your support team may take longer to accept your diagnosis and may take time to catch up. Do your best to communicate your thought process and be prepared to be patient with others as they won't process the news, options, and treatment plan as quickly as you.

Belief

People exceptionally talented in the Belief theme have certain core values that are unchanging. These values provide direction and a strong sense of purpose.

> My friend died of breast cancer while trying to make a difference and trying to end breast cancer. We can't be a nation of people who just sit and let problems pass them by. You have to be political about it if you want to save lives.
>
> —Kristin, breast cancer survivor

You have certain core values that are enduring. These values vary from one person to another, but typically, having strong Belief causes you to be altruistic, even spiritual, and to value responsibility and high ethics—both in yourself and others. These core values give your life meaning and satisfaction, and they affect your behaviors and decisions. Your values give you direction and guide you through the temptations and distractions of life toward a consistent set of priorities. This consistency is the foundation for all your relationships. Your Belief makes you easy to trust. Your friends call you dependable. They know where you stand. In your view, success is more than money and prestige. Guided by your Belief theme, your work must be meaningful and fit with your values; it must matter to you. And it will matter only if it gives you the chance to live out your values.

Characteristics of Those with Belief Talents

Certain	Unchanging	Passionate	Self-sacrificing
Stable	Principled	Committed	

Cancer Connection

People with the strength of Belief are committed to their core values and take their purpose or mission seriously. You may be crystal clear on your guiding principles that drive the direction of your life and decisions, or you may be refining, revisiting, and still gaining clarity. No matter where you are in your certainty, your cancer diagnosis may rattle you a bit. There is not an absolute when it comes to how cancer will impact your direction. Some cancer survivors double down on the things they were focusing on prior to their diagnosis. Others may do a 180 and shift their attention to different arenas or relationships. Regardless of the impact of your diagnosis, you will still take life seriously and maintain a strong commitment to ethical causes and serving others.

Kristin Teig Torres is a 15-year breast cancer survivor, a mother of two, an incredible actress in community productions, and a fundraising adviser. Kristin dug into advocacy work in honor of her friend, Anne Christensen Doyle, who passed away from breast cancer. This loss impacted her tremendously, and she felt like she owed it to her friend to get involved and be a strong voice in the fight for research dollars and policies. In an interview with the *Waterloo-Cedar Falls Courier* Kristin said, "She died trying to make a difference and trying to end breast cancer, so I went to my first National Breast Cancer Coalition leadership summit the year after she died. We can't be a nation of people who just sit and let problems pass them by."[27]

---

[27] Crippes, C. (September 2016) "Torres Focuses on Advocacy, Education to End Breast Cancer," *The Courier*. Available at: https://wcfcourier.com/news/local/torres-focuses-on-advocacy-education-to-end-breast-cancer/article_d8fe0a7b-cd53-538d-8ede-39cbefb125cb.html.

In speaking with Kristin, I was struck by the sheer amount of time she has devoted to advocacy work in over a decade. She serves on the local Beyond Pink TEAM's Advocacy Committee and completed the National Breast Cancer Coalition's Project LEAD, a premier science training program for advocates. She is relentless in her commitment to meeting with our state senators and representatives. I've joined Kristin and other local advocates in Washington, D.C., twice, and when I asked more about this drive and devotion, Kristin passionately replied, "You have to be political about it if you want to save lives." That is the epitome of a person with the Belief strength selflessly putting their passion and conviction in motion toward the fight to end cancer. Kristin has clearly honored and developed her Belief strength during the thousands of hours she has committed toward ending breast cancer.

My own Belief strength fueled me to use this awful diagnosis to eventually help others. It was this passion that drove me to document my thoughts, questions, and challenges as I endured chemotherapy, surgery, and recovery. It was this strength that pushed me to dig deeper into Gallup's research, interview other cancer survivors, and make good on my gut feeling to write this book. Although I could have dismissed that instinct as a coping mechanism or a delusional thought, I knew all along that I would follow through, no matter how much procrastination or how many hurdles I faced along the way.

Since receiving my diagnosis, I have dabbled in a few different areas of cancer volunteering, mentoring, and advocacy work. Serving with my husband as a member of the American Cancer Society's Iowa board of directors and the American Cancer Society Cancer Action Network (ACS CAN) has been extremely rewarding. ACS CAN "advocates for evidence-based public policies to reduce the cancer burden for everyone."[28] I feel energized and purposeful when using my Belief strength to meet with elected officials for advocacy work, host and participate in fundraisers, and raise awareness in our community about cancer statistics

---

28 American Cancer Society Cancer Action Network. Available at: https://www.fightcancer.org/about.

and programs. Spending time with my family is important to me, and we have enjoyed participating in the local Relay for Life event, the Coaches vs. Cancer gala, and the Charity Golf Classic. We love the overlap of these events with golf and basketball and are participating out of interest and not obligation. This is an important distinction to make for cancer survivors and to be sure you are effectively tapping into your Belief strength.

Cancer Considerations

Put your health and treatment first
After hearing your diagnosis, you may be looking externally for ways to make a difference. This is natural for people with the Belief strength, but prioritization is critical right now. Spend time understanding your care options and how this will impact your life in the months or years going forward. Put your health and treatment first, and opportunities to give back and serve can follow.

Review your core values
Spend time examining or revisiting your personal core values. What are the most important considerations and principles you follow in living your life? A few examples of values are achievement, adventure, creativity, fairness, faith, or service. You will be faced with dozens, if not hundreds, of important decisions in the weeks and months ahead. As you consider your options and weigh the pros and cons of different choices, do a quick alignment check with your values. If you find yourself overwhelmed with certain decisions, check in with yourself on the principles you hold closest and do your best to align your decision-making with your values.

There are values card sorts or worksheets available online, some free and others at a nominal cost. If you are interested in exploring Gallup's Values cards, see Resources for Surviving Cancer with Your Strengths (page 335).

Others can help move your mission forward
Take time to reflect on how you've inspired others in your life. Receive and soak in that goodness. Be open to their offers to help you as they may see this as a time to repay you for your past good deeds and kindnesses. You have a gift in providing others with clarity and conviction, so work to anticipate where you may need assistance in fulfilling your commitments. These may be focused on your career, your family, your faith organization, or your community. Can somebody else take some steps to move your mission or interests forward?

Who needs you most?
Hearing the news of your diagnosis can be a life-altering experience. With your Belief talents, you are likely family-oriented, others-oriented, and committed to these relationships. Are there activities or causes you can engage in collectively? Are there ways you'd like to spend your time effectively with family members? Now is a great time to do a time audit. Ensure you are aligning your core values with where you are spending your precious time and who gets to enjoy that time with you.

Evaluate your commitments
You are likely involved in community organizations or initiatives, whether as a visionary, organizer, volunteer, or participant. Evaluate if you need to see progress in those areas while you endure treatment or if a coasting speed works for now. Will continuing these efforts fuel your Belief talents or does anything need to be altered or tabled for the time being? For example, are there tasks you can take on virtually when your energy or immunity is down? If you are leading a committee, is it possible to switch roles and participate as a member, rather than the leader, for the short term? Work to develop a backup plan for your participation levels while in treatment, if possible, with the goal of resuming activities upon recovery.

Attend to what fuels your fire
As you learn more about your diagnosis and prognosis, lean on your Belief talents for fuel to help you continue living your purpose and focusing on

your values and mission. Belief is often a motor that drives you and fuels your fire, so zero in on this when you need to improve your energy levels and reinvigorate your productivity.

Your purpose and values may not lead you toward civic, political, or leadership roles. But do listen closely to what fuels your fire. It may be a cause, a mission, a project, or an individual you feel passionate about helping or serving. Your Belief strength could also set you up to be a passionate committee member for cancer-related causes, an advocate for health policy improvements, or an inspiring mentor for newly diagnosed cancer survivors. Audit your energy levels and determine what you can put toward this arena. This work could drain most people and feel like a *nice to do,* but it could energize you and be closer to a *must do.*

Here is an example of my neighbor and one of my breast cancer mentors, Sharon, who had Belief as a top strength. Despite 12 years living with Stage 4 metastatic breast cancer and the numerous health challenges it created for her, Sharon elected to run for city council. Concerned friends tried to talk her out of it, given her age and health challenges, but Sharon's commitment to her purpose propelled her forward. Her first campaign message stated, "During the weeks leading up to the election, I hope you will learn more about my love for Waterloo, my core values, and why I believe my experience makes me uniquely qualified for this position." She made significant contributions during her four years before opting not to run again with a statement that said, "We are on the brink of achieving great things, but I do not have the energy that Waterloo citizens deserve to maintain a front-row seat."

Sharon's beautiful obituary, written by her twin daughters, read "Sharon was a quintessential community builder and lived out this purpose in her professional and personal life. She had the privilege of being involved in over 75 organizations and associations, often taking on a leadership role, including her 25 years as Executive Director at an association of local governments."

I am so thankful for Sharon's friendship, leadership, and cancer mentorship. Miss you, neighbor.

Cancer Cautions

Cancer may be only a detour
Cancer does not need to become your purpose. Given your passion and energy around important causes, you may feel led or inspired to go all in with an organization or a mission related to this disease. In fact, those close to you may even have ideas and suggestions given how they've witnessed your mission-driven talents prior to your diagnosis. Keep in mind your purpose may have been clearly defined long before you received a cancer diagnosis, and it's perfectly fine for this disease to be only a detour, not your new course. The decision is yours.

Marshal your resources wisely
Cancer may lead to fatigue and less energy. Evaluate how and where you're spending your time serving others as you plan your days and weeks. For example, if you are involved in committees, serve on a board, or volunteer within the community, each activity should be examined to determine if it remains on your list as you move through your diagnosis, treatment, and recovery. The advice is not to stop serving or making an impact; however, weigh your energy expenditures wisely as your resources will be depleted.

Bring others along with you
Perhaps there have been times in your life where people have perceived you as stubborn or set in your ways. Instead, you may have been so clearly guided and driven by your values this could have come off as intolerance or closed-mindedness. I know people thought I was nuts when in between my first and second chemotherapies, I declared I was going to write a book to help cancer survivors. Many recommended that I should wait until I finished treatment to decide if that was still a good idea or something I even cared about doing. In the seven years it took me to finish the book, I sometimes laughed—they may have been right! But I honestly knew I would do it all along, no matter how valid anyone's feedback was to reconsider my plan. Having the Belief strength can inspire

others to act. Once you've determined your direction, make sure you bring others along with your energy and enthusiasm.

Command

People exceptionally talented in the Command theme have presence. They can take control of a situation and make decisions.

> Clear is kind.
> Unclear is unkind.
>
> —Dr. Brené Brown,
> research professor
> and New York Times
> bestselling author

Command leads you to take charge. Unlike some people, you feel no discomfort imposing your views on others. On the contrary, once you form your opinion, you need to share it with others. Once you set a goal, you feel restless until you have aligned others with you. You are not afraid of confrontation; rather, you believe that confrontation is the first step toward resolution. Others may avoid facing up to life's unpleasantness, but you feel compelled to present the truth, no matter how unpleasant it may be. You need things to be clear between people, and you challenge others to be realistic and honest. You push them to take risks. You may even intimidate them. And while some may resent this and consider you opinionated, they often willingly hand you the reins. People are drawn to those who take a stand and who can persuade them to move in a certain direction. Because of your talents, people will be drawn to you. You have presence. You have Command.

Characteristics of Those with Command Talents

Decisive	Driven	Challenging	Assertive
Opinionated	Strong-willed	Clarifying	Persuasive
Intimidating	Controlling	Imposing	Candid

Cancer Connection

You are naturally a courageous fighter. While cancer may be the toughest challenge you've faced in your lifetime, you are wired to move through this with more confidence and assertiveness than most. Although there may be days ahead containing medical setbacks, physical challenges, or emotional uncertainty, you have always been up for a challenge. If each strength had a theme song, Billy Ocean's 1985 hit "When the Going Gets Tough, the Tough Get Going" may be a perfect fit for Command. Summon your inner courage and strength to keep you moving forward with clarity and confidence.

Maika Leibbrandt, former Gallup Senior Consultant, shares on the Gallup Access Command online training module, "I think about Command as being the anchor, the navigator, and the captain. It can keep us grounded, help us move, or tell us more out loud what we need to be doing. There's a beauty to Command that's all about truth."[29] What powerful image or analogy could help you draw on this strength and guide you through your cancer experience? What truth about your health do you need to share with others?

You have a natural talent for decisiveness. Your cancer diagnosis will present you with the opportunity to make hundreds of decisions, and your Command strength will give you an edge as you consider all your options. There are typically multiple locations, physicians, and treatment

---

29 Gallup CliftonStrengths, "Learn About the Science and Validity of CliftonStrengths." Available at: https://www.gallup.com/cliftonstrengths/en/252176/command-learning-love-talent-themes.aspx.

options to evaluate. Your natural certainty will help you navigate this process. Embrace your natural decisiveness and share your talent with those who join you on your cancer journey. Many people may want nothing more than to help you out, so they'll jump through hoops to drive you to chemotherapy, water your flowers, and take your kids for ice cream. Yet when it comes time to pick a parking place at the hospital or decide where to grab lunch afterward, arguably the simplest of decisions, they'll probably still need you to make the final call. Because that's the value you've shared so beautifully with others all these years.

Given that Command is statistically one of the rarest strengths globally, according to Gallup, your medical care team may be surprised by your willingness to challenge them with your thoughts and questions, and your ability to ask for and embrace truth. Depending on their strengths and expertise, they may find this talent of yours refreshing. Many medical professionals are fact-based, objective, and analytical by nature. Whereas people are often intimidated by your assertiveness, your medical team may relish your desire for clarity. My good friend and Australia-based Gallup-Certified Strengths Coach, Charlotte Blair, experienced a horse-riding accident years ago breaking seven ribs and puncturing her lung. As she was wheeled into the operating room and introduced to her surgeon she said, "You had better be good, Benjamin," in her playful yet persuasive British accent. Charlotte didn't see him again until her six-week checkup and he reminded her of what she said. He handed her his business card, smiled, and suggested she contact him directly if she had any problems.

Charlotte explained, "A few weeks later I was experiencing some significant discomfort and was worried a screw had become dislodged. I tried to book in for an appointment but was told his schedule was full and he couldn't see me for a week. People with Command are known for pushing back, so I emailed him directly and Dr. Benjamin told me to come in the next morning at 9 a.m." This is a perfect example of how being direct is in your favor right now.

If your provider is defensive, instead of impressed like Dr. Benjamin, explain that you are typically the one in control of challenging situations and it's helpful for you to have honest answers to even the most difficult of questions. Remember too that although you may not be an oncologist or an expert on cancer, you are always in the driver's seat when it comes to your own health and well-being, and your assertiveness is a wonderful strength to use.

Cancer Considerations

Cut to the chase
You have a strength for honesty and truthfulness. You are often the person who will say the thing that others are thinking but won't say. Use your ability to cut to the chase at doctor's appointments, family discussions, and conversations with those providing you support.

Tell people what you need and when you need it. Even if you can't make it work, you will feel in control. One breast cancer survivor and business executive shared that it was important for her to "move the ball fast and that cancer didn't stop me." She continued to go to her son's games and travel for work. Diane shared that she had an important work trip in San Francisco approaching. Her doctor advised her to stay home since she needed to have shots administered during that timeframe. Diane said, "I'm NOT not doing things because I have to take shots. Figure out another way." She ended up going on the trip and having a nurse give her the injections during a break from her meetings.

Share your approach for facing reality
You have a knack for facing reality, including awful situations, head on. Although cancer is a scary diagnosis, you can still move through it with confidence. You may notice that people around you are slower to catch up with this mindset. Be prepared to have direct conversations with those who need to understand your approach and bring them along with you, as you have done in the past. Once they can accept the truth of your health challenge, they will find your candidness and honesty moving and refreshing.

Engage in advocacy

Consider using your voice, your directness, and your persuasive talents in an advocacy role. You may be willing to challenge authority or the status quo, which is a valuable skillset in activism. Your strong voice can impact public policy decisions related to healthcare, insurance, research funding, environmental contaminants, and disparities and inequities in medical outcomes. Persuading others in the political arena is an extraordinary and rare quality.

Set the tone

Possessing the strength of Command provides you with a need for emotional clarity. Others may look to you for how to respond to this shocking news and intimidating treatment steps. Those who know you best have likely turned to you for guidance and support over the years. Although you are now the patient, you can still set the tone for the emotional vibe you'd like to feel from your supporters. You might share something like, "I know this is a surprise, but I don't want you to stay angry for long. I was at first, but now I am ready to begin my cancer treatment and heal. I'd love it if you could join me in moving forward."

Cancer Cautions

Work out what's in your control

A cancer diagnosis is unsettling to everybody regardless of their strengths. You are naturally wired to control situations with your strong presence. There are many aspects of cancer that you will not be able to control, such as your tumors or white blood cell counts. Analyze what aspects of your cancer experience you can impact, what portions you can directly control, and let those other pieces go. This is not an act of giving up. It is an act of getting clarity on where your power lies.

Understand there will be ambiguity
As you progress through your treatment plan and recovery, there may be medical gray areas. You don't have much of a tolerance for ambiguity in your life but be prepared for uncertainty in your cancer experience. For example, if you seek a second or third opinion, different healthcare providers may offer different treatments options. You may have to evaluate incomplete information and conflicting insights and make the decision that is best for you with what you know at that time.

Engage your medical team in your decision-making
You are an excellent decision-maker. When it comes to decisions related to your cancer treatment plan and related health decisions, make sure you are evaluating sufficient facts and information before deciding. Ask your most trusted supporters and members of your medical team, "I'm leaning toward this decision. What am I missing or what haven't I considered?" This open-ended question will either validate that you've thought through the alternatives or allow them to share additional facts or resources. You want to make sure your decisiveness is a benefit to you.

Communication

People exceptionally talented in the Communication theme generally find it easy to put their thoughts into words. They are good conversationalists and presenters.

During an overwhelming and stressful time of navigating a cancer diagnosis and treatment, having a dedicated notebook helps feed your need for clarity with your strength of Communication.

—Ali, caregiver for her father

You have a natural ability to explain, describe, speak in public, and write. You need to bring ideas to life—to energize them, to make them exciting and vivid. Using the power of words, you animate ideas with images, examples, and metaphors. You create compelling stories and practice telling them. You believe that most people have a very short attention span because they are constantly bombarded with information. But you want to direct their attention toward you, capture it, and lock it in. You want your message to survive. This is what drives your hunt for the perfect phrase. This is what draws you to dramatic language and powerful word combinations. This is why people like to listen to you. Your words grab their interest, sharpen their world and inspire them.

Characteristics of Those with Communication Talents

Talkative	Verbal	Interactive
Presenting	Transparent	Conversational
Entertaining	Captivating	Expressive

Cancer Connection

You are known for your words and your ability to connect with people through how you communicate. Some people with Communication as a strength are great storytellers, writers, conversationalists, and even listeners. Many people with this strength feel that events don't seem real until they've had a chance to share them out loud. They say that talking through experiences, information, or emotions is how they process things best. Reflect on your strength of Communication and how it's allowed you to shine in the past. Think about specific examples and dig deeper with a few questions. Where are you when you get the most energized through communication? Who are some of your favorite people to spend time with in conversation? Purposely work to create these special connections in these preferred locations. If you love telling stories, pick up the phone and call a friend. If you love writing, grab a notepad or your computer and head to a cozy coffee shop.

As you go through your cancer experience, being in communication with others will be important to you. Your health may impact your energy levels and decrease the amount of face-to-face time you're able to spend with others. Remain open to other types of connecting such as phone calls, text messages, or social media as these forms of communication may still fill your tank.

You may have a knack for picking just the right word or sharing an expression that creates an *aha* moment in the room. So, if the precision of the words related to your diagnosis is important to you, let others know so you can help shape and control that messaging. You may want people to know that you have a specific form of melanoma and what makes that unique. You may want people to understand that you have Stage 0 cancer and that your survival rate is 95%. Tara is a breast cancer survivor and shared, "We need to learn to speak in parts. Saying, 'I have breast cancer in my right breast' is different from saying 'I have cancer.'" Tara continued by saying, "I don't want cancer to be a journey. I want it to be a project that has a start and an end. That has been an interesting discovery. Language is so powerful." When it comes to your health messaging, you can play a variety of roles from brand strategist to content creator to editor to announcer.

Communication of a cancer diagnosis can be done however it feels best to you. There are so many different and equally acceptable ways to share your diagnosis and future health updates. If it feels right to you, reach out to people to talk about your diagnosis, treatment, and survivorship. If you want people to hear your voice, make the phone calls. If you want them to hear it by phone, but you don't have the time or energy to spend making all the calls, ask a loved one to help. If you prefer to fire off a text, people can handle receiving your health information over text. Some cancer survivors immediately take to social media to share the life altering news; others never share it with anyone.

For those of you with the strength of Communication, you will have an advantage in working through who to tell, when to tell, and how to do it. Given your gift for gab, once you've made these decisions, delivering the message may be the easier part. You likely feel comfortable chatting with people, sharing stories, and ensuring that your message is understood. Although the update you're about to share with people is a difficult one to digest, you will deliver it like a natural.

Cancer Considerations

Be open to another perspective
Holly, a Stage 0 breast cancer survivor with the Communication strength, passionately explained the importance of seeking a second opinion. The

breast surgeon at her local cancer center performed an excisional biopsy on an area of concern one year prior to her diagnosis. She trusted him and felt confident in his abilities when she was faced with the decision between a lumpectomy and mastectomy just one year later.

While she initially planned to proceed with him for her double mastectomy surgery, her mom encouraged her to make one more phone call. Bev connected her daughter with a former community member, breast cancer survivor, and nurse navigator at another cancer center in the state. Although she resisted the idea of getting a second opinion at first, Holly took her lovely 85-year-old mom's advice and reached out to the local connection. This conversation was a pivotal point of Holly's cancer experience and decision-making process.

She shared, "For me, it was such a game changer to get a second opinion. I ended up moving my entire care two hours south from where we live. It was the best decision I made in my cancer journey." She expanded, "Even if you feel comfortable with your initial provider and inclined to stay with them for continuity of care, getting a second opinion allows you to explore other options and gain clarity." Additionally, Holly encourages cancer survivors to trust their instincts. She said, "If you're frustrated by delays or the pace of care, use that as a prompt to seek another opinion."

Even if you stick with your initial plan, getting another perspective helps ensure you are making the most informed decision for you personally, as every treatment plan is individualized.

Make a plan to share updates

As your treatment progresses, it's wise to have a plan for sharing updates. Given your knack for conversation, you may prefer for people to hear updates firsthand from you. It may boost your energy to share written and verbal progress with those concerned. You are the director of this show, and if you want the microphone in your hand, then it's all yours.

Many cancer survivors create an online source of updates, whether it's through email, social media platforms, or a nonprofit website like CaringBridge.[30] Although I opted to share periodic updates by text and

---

30 CaringBridge: https://www.caringbridge.org.

on Facebook, CaringBridge is currently the most used free website for health updates. Over 240,000 people use this private communications platform daily in 244 countries and territories, and more than one million pages have been created since 1997. It allows you or a trusted loved one to share journal entries, photos, and ways for people to help such as buying groceries or providing meals.

Appoint a press secretary
Who can be your press secretary when you're too tired to talk, but want your message shared? For example, if surgery is part of your treatment plan, allocate somebody to communicate how things went with your desired list of friends and loved ones. You can contribute to the message or review it before they hit *Send*, but don't feel the pressure to write your own updates.

Who needs to know what?
Consider creating levels of access to your time and energy, like the levels of seating at an arena for a concert. Your inner circle is likely in the VIP section and may even have backstage passes to spend more time with you. Other friends or colleagues may be in the upper level. They're in the arena, but they may not have the clearest view or see and hear every move.

Is anyone on your "Do not call" list? That may sound harsh, but some well-intentioned people can exhaust cancer survivors and may not need a ticket, so to speak. It is critically important for you to understand how various people impact your energy and emotions and allow access accordingly. Make sure those nearest to you are also aware of your preferences.

Talking with the right people
If you'd like additional medical support for discussing your health, contact a therapist, oncology psychologist, or another professional your institution recommends. If you find value in talking with other cancer survivors, consider attending a support group. Some organizations even provide 1:1 support with a trained volunteer, such as the American

Cancer Society CARES™ (Community Access to Resources, Education, and Support) mobile app.[31]

About five weeks into my breast cancer diagnosis, my breast cancer mentor and new friend, Sarah, and I were having lunch together. She was on her second bout with breast cancer and bluntly shared that you don't want cancer to return. While hers was still contained to her breast, she told me about another woman whose breast cancer had metastasized to her brain. Sarah's description of metastasis, and prognosis of "If it spreads, you're screwed," knocked the wind out of me. I had been so focused on the current state of my cancer treatment plan that I hadn't given much thought to the reality that it could return someday. Sarah's colorful language sent me into a tailspin of worry, fear, and anxiety and I spent the entire afternoon curled up in the recliner.

At my next appointment, I questioned my oncologist about recurrence. She shared the percentage odds of recurrence, and I wasn't anywhere close to prepared for the number to be that high. She sensed the fear in my facial expression and quickly offered to refer me to an oncology psychologist. After two sessions with him, I felt better about the data, able to manage my worry and move forward. It was a relief to voice my concerns to a neutral party who was an expert in the cancer and psychology arena. He didn't dismiss my worry, like a friend or family member may nervously do. Instead, he acknowledged that fear of recurrence is a real thing for survivors and discussed approaches to managing fear and worry productively.

If your time and financial or healthcare insurance resources allow, talking concerns through with an expert can reduce your stress and anxiety and is worth the investment. You have plenty to talk about related to your cancer diagnosis and doing that with an expert will meet your needs of being heard and processing this challenge verbally. Their words may energize you and provide new cancer-related terms and expressions that capture your thoughts and emotions.

---

31 ACS CARES™, American Cancer Society. Available at: https://www.cancer.org/support-programs-and-services/acs-cares.html.

You write your own scripts

You may be known as an entertainer, a storyteller, or even a comedian. You get to control when you tell the stories, how many details you share, and if any of your explanations contain humor. If it's cathartic for you to laugh along the way, go for it. If you find renewed energy and strength through blogging, journaling, or posting to social media, have at it.

As you pick and choose what stories to tell, when to tell them, and how to share them, keep in mind that even entertainers take vacations. Don't feel pressure from your audience to get onstage, online, or on the phone. You're the screenwriter, the actor, and the director. You control if, and when, to say, "Action!"

Chance encounters

Cancer centers are often very peaceful and comforting environments. It may give you a boost to talk with the healthcare employees, other patients, and those in the waiting rooms and hallways. Your ease with words and friendly bantering may be "just what the doctor ordered" for other cancer survivors and their concerned loved ones. If you sense that people are drawn toward being in conversation and it feels energizing to you, enjoy the connection.

Do be aware, especially early in your cancer experience, that not everybody has this strength of yours and may prefer silence over small talk. A cancer center is full of varied emotions and energy levels and your Communication strength will help you navigate it appropriately.

If you're a writer, write!

Prior to receiving your cancer diagnosis, if writing was a source of energy for you, a hobby, or even a passion, don't stop now. You don't have to share anything you write—in fact, you may need to keep your writing to yourself, at least for now, but please be sure to give yourself the space to write to express yourself if you find it energizing. And if you want to share your writing about your cancer experience with others, that's wonderful. But please don't pressure yourself to become a bestselling author while you're sick from chemo or in pain from radiation. Sharing in small ways can be enough right now—maybe an email about your treatment with a few close friends, or a personal Facebook group, private blog, or on a reputable cancer-related platform. For now, think about what serves you best. Worry less about where your words live and more about how they help you come alive along the way.

Share your experience
If you're interested in sharing your cancer experience when you're further along in the process, your Communication strength will be very valuable. You can leverage this talent through presentations, writing, conversing, or persuading. Opportunities include mentoring newly diagnosed cancer survivors, writing articles, sharing your story publicly, engaging in advocacy work, or fundraising for a cancer organization. Pull in your best thought partner, whether that is your partner, friend, coach, or another cancer survivor. Schedule time with this trusted person to rehearse your thoughts before sharing them more broadly.

Cancer Cautions

Take your time
People have become accustomed to you having just the right words for any situation. This may be a time where you're not sure what to say, how to say it, or whether to say it. If you'd like to provide a health update, you have full permission to say you're not sure what to say or that you don't have all the information. People have valued and trusted how you've communicated over the years. They will trust you on this one too.

Not everyone is a gifted communicator
Many people are not as thoughtful and gifted with words as you. This may include some of your closest supporters, friends, and family, which can lead to some awkward exchanges like "My aunt had ovarian cancer too. She didn't make it, but I know you're going to beat it." Crickets.

And it may include your oncologist, radiologist, surgeon, and other members of your care team. There may be times when the medical information presented to you is not as clear as you'd prefer, so be prepared to ask clarifying questions. Given your knack for analogies and stories, you may be able to articulate something more vividly than your care team. Make sure you leave appointments with all the information you need to accurately understand and repeat what you heard.

Ali shared that it was helpful to carry a dedicated notebook to her dad's appointments during the 10 years he was being treated for his brain tumors. Her dad was a farmer and called the notebook his "vet book." She said, "My mom and I took it to every appointment and were responsible for making note of what we learned. This was immensely helpful to refer back to later when we were sharing updates with my sisters or if we had a discrepancy in what we each remembered from the appointment." Ali added that during an overwhelming and stressful time of navigating a cancer diagnosis and treatment, having these notes helps feed your need for clarity with your strength of Communication.

Plan your conversations with your medical team
If you are a natural conversationalist and love to talk, you may enjoy visiting with your healthcare team members and providers. While that is certainly a positive, keep in mind that they may have a limited amount of time to spend with you. Prioritize your talking points and questions to address top areas of concern, confusion, and curiosity. Ensure you are getting all your questions answered and you have clarity about your next steps before branching into other topics. It's always advisable to have somebody join you for appointments. Ask them to help you make a list of questions in rank order, take notes of the responses, and stay on track during your appointments.

Competition

People exceptionally talented in the Competition theme measure their progress against the performance of others. They love contests and need to win.

Competition is rooted in comparison. When you look at the world, you are instinctively aware of other people's performance. It is your ultimate benchmark. No matter how hard you try, no matter how worthy your intentions, if you reach your goal but do not outperform your peers, the achievement feels hollow. You like measurement because it makes it easier to compare. If you can compare, you can compete. If you can compete, you can win. And when you win, there is no feeling quite like it. You like other competitors because they invigorate you. You like contests because they must produce a winner. You particularly like contests when you know you have an advantage, and you will avoid contests when winning seems unlikely. You don't compete for the fun of competing—you compete to win.

Cancer can take away all of my physical abilities. It cannot touch my mind, it cannot touch my heart, and it cannot touch my soul. And those three things are going to carry on forever.

—Jim Volvano (1946–1993), basketball coach, broadcaster, and founder of the V Foundation

Characteristics of Those with Competition Talents

Scorekeeping   Winning   Aspiring
Intense   Comparing   Measuring
Driven   Selective

Cancer Connection

You need metrics, measurements, and benchmarks to know where you stand. Let's face it. You play to win. If there's a contest, race, or a chance for victory, you're in. You've faced many opponents in your lifetime, some aware and others oblivious they were your rival. You're at your best when you can compare your performance to something or someone else. You are motivated to win and be the best. Winning brings emotions with it, feelings you cannot escape. The pain of defeat is a passenger you carry with you long after others have moved on. Similarly, the power boost of a win can fuel you, elevating your lived experience to higher places than others may reach.

While many patients struggle with resiliency and maintaining a healthy mindset through cancer, you have an edge here. You feel best when you're competing and comparing, so find something you can count and track to monitor your fight. Whereas those with Competition lower on their list of strengths may struggle with the "fight cancer" mentality, you thrive as long as you can measure your progress against something external. Your champion's mindset is not just about thinking differently. It's best when translated into action, and your experience overcoming hardship on the road to victory will be a unique advantage for you.

A tremendous amount of marketing and messaging around cancer, in the United States at least, is centered around the metaphor of fighting. The words are punchy and feisty like "Crush Cancer!" "Nobody Fights Alone!" and "Kick cancer's a*s!" For some, these words fall flat and don't serve as an adrenaline boost. For someone like you who is innately competitive, they just might be speaking your language and fire you up along the way.

Sarah is the first survivor I spoke to hours after my breast cancer diagnosis. I didn't know Sarah prior to that horrible day, but she is now a friend and my cancer mentor, one of the gifts to come out of this nightmare. She is a marketing executive, mother to three, a breast cancer advocate, and a philanthropist who casually raised one million dollars for an inclusive park in our community. In the throes of treatment, Sarah found something to compete against—her own time. During our first lunch, Sarah shared that she made some of her medical decisions based on how much time various treatment options would take her away from work. For example, she opted for double dosage amounts of chemotherapy to reduce the number of infusions she'd need. Blown away by her tenacity and drive, I asked Sarah how many vacation days she used to balance work, family life, and treatments. I'll never forget her response. Sarah stopped eating her salad, looked me squarely in the eye, and confidently replied, "Cancer's not getting any of my PTO [paid time off]." Sure enough, one of Sarah's top strengths is Competition, and seeing cancer as her opposition was a motivator for her.

Cancer Considerations

Surround yourself with motivation
Curate your Champion's Circle, a motivating environment around you for what you see and hear. Do you have some favorite quotes, or have you heard new ones related to cancer as something to beat? Consider displaying them where you can see them as a daily reminder to draw on your desire to win.

Create a playlist
What's your favorite music to get your blood flowing? These popular anthems may spark some ideas for you: "Eye of the Tiger" by Survivor for *Rocky III,* "Fight Song" by Rachel Platten, "Girl on Fire" by Alicia Keys, "Don't Stop Me Now" by Queen, or "All I Do Is Win" by DJ Khaled. Pump

up whatever jams fuel your inner warrior in your moments of fatigue, frustration, or restlessness. Create a playlist to boost your competitive spirit.

Find a like-minded soul

Game recognizes game. Find a cancer survivor who approached the disease in a competitive way. This could be a friend, relative, community member, or a famous person. Explore what made their cancer experience unique and admirable by talking with them or reading about them in books or online. What fierce approach or attitude did they bring to cancer that you'd like to emulate? How would you compare your approach to theirs?

Just a few months before college basketball coach Jim Valvano passed away from metastatic adenocarcinoma, he shared an iconic speech at the Excellence in Sports Performance Yearly Awards Event (the ESPYs) famously saying, "Don't give up, don't ever give up." During his speech, he announced the creation of the V Foundation for Cancer Research with a singular mission: to achieve Victory over Cancer®.

To date, the foundation that he, and the sports entertainment and news network ESPN, founded has raised over $353 million in grants for cancer research. Coach Valvano's final words of his famous 10-minute speech demonstrated his competitive spirit as he closed by saying, "Cancer can take away all of my physical abilities. It cannot touch my mind, it cannot touch my heart, and it cannot touch my soul. And those three things are going to carry on forever."[32]

Define your wins

Share your motivation to compete with your medical team. Encourage them not to hide external comparisons or stories from you. In fact, ask them how success can be determined for your unique situation, and how others have succeeded. Look for which practices they have noticed give people "an edge" for their diagnosis. Ask them what above and beyond healing would look like for a patient with your type of cancer. You are willing to put in the work if that will increase your odds for successful treatment outcomes.

---

32 Watch Coach Valvano's speech at: https://www.v.org/jim-valvano.

Create goals with metrics
Find something to count and rank. What numbers do you want to meet or beat? This could be a daily number of steps taken, vegetables eaten, minutes read, or meditation sessions completed. Have fun with these challenges and create contests that benefit your health and satisfy your constant internal scorekeeper. Keep striving to hit those goals, track your success, and celebrate your wins.

Cancer Cautions

Other people are not competing with you
Reminder: You are not trying to beat all the other cancer patients you meet. Whether you meet them in the waiting rooms or through introductions from friends and family, keep in mind that they are on your team. These people are not opponents to measure your cancer "performance" against. They may not have, or need, the same benchmarks as you to determine what a win looks like. See them as teammates and friends.

Nurture your need to compete
Don't ditch all competitive endeavors in an effort to streamline your strengths at only fighting cancer. You will show up even stronger during your treatment and recovery if you are active in outside competitions. Find a challenge that gets you a legitimate win, even if it has seemingly nothing to do with hospitals or healthcare.

Pushing yourself isn't always a win
You love a good challenge, and it will be important for you to keep that intense drive. Be careful not to sacrifice your health or ignore your doctor's advice. Facing difficult side effects or a setback with your health often leads to delays in your cancer treatment. Balance your need to push yourself harder than most people with the reality that your immunity is down and your body needs rest.

Connectedness

People exceptionally talented in the Connectedness theme believe everything is linked and that there are few coincidences. For them, everything happens for a reason.

> I felt like I was part of a community of people across time who have had or will have cancer, and I felt solidarity with them.
>
> —Mary Sue, breast cancer survivor

Things happen for a reason—you feel it deep in your soul. You know we're all connected in some way. Yes, we have free will, and we're responsible for our own choices. But even so, we're part of something much bigger. You're certain of the oneness of humanity. Some might call it the collective unconscious, spirit, or life force. Whatever words resonate with you, understanding that we're not isolated from one another gives you strength—and it comes with certain responsibilities. If we're all part of a greater whole, then hurting others ultimately means hurting ourselves. Exploiting our communities means exploiting ourselves. These beliefs shape your values. You are considerate, caring, and accepting. You build bridges between people from different cultures and backgrounds. You reassure others that there's a purpose beyond the routine of daily life. The details of your faith may be influenced by your upbringing and culture, but your faith is steadfast nonetheless. It sustains you and helps you navigate the mysteries of life with confidence and grace.

Characteristics of Those with Connectedness Talents

Integrating	Spiritual	Perceptive
Philosophic	Listening	Seeking
Comforting	Mystical	Counseling

Cancer Connection

You are likely an intuitive person. Your strength of Connectedness gives you great perspective as you think a lot about how people, places, or events are interconnected. As you go through your cancer experience, you may interact with people from multiple specialties in the healthcare system. While their areas of expertise are specialized, you will view these professionals and seemingly separate departments as all part of one team, your care team. You may take a more holistic or integrative approach to how you think about, and possibly even treat, your cancer because of your strength of Connectedness. Andrea shared:

> Connectedness can be used as a filter when choosing the right healthcare providers. I had the good fortune and blessing of getting the best care through Memorial Sloan Kettering (MSK) in New York City. The value and importance I place on a connected culture, which MSK demonstrates in practice and spirit, were very influential in how I approached my diagnosis, treatment, and recovery. The team and the trusted relationships I built at MSK provided me with the hope and faith that I needed to navigate my journey successfully.

Stay dialed in to your intuitive thoughts and feelings and challenge yourself to share these impressions with others. Depending on what you are sensing, this might mean sharing ideas, questions, or even messages of hope or faith with your medical team, your family, or other cancer survivors you connect with along the way. Regardless of the audience, they may not grasp what you're sharing. Connectedness is a unique strength that may provide you with ideas and answers that are difficult to explain with data, proof, or anything that others can see. That's okay—let yourself benefit from the intuitive connections you make.

I spoke with Mary Sue Ingraham, a breast cancer survivor, executive coach, and longtime Gallup-Certified Strengths Coach, about her diagnosis and treatment experience. She shared:

> From the very beginning, I had a bigger perspective on it. There is a global empathy tied to Connectedness that gives me an aerial perspective of the past, present, and future and how they connect. I felt like I was part of a community of people across time who have had or will have cancer, and I felt solidarity with them. Early on, I realized I would never again be in the metaphorical river of "she never had cancer," and that for the rest of my life this would be part of my story. I pictured that I was now on a white-water river, one I'd never navigated before. The river was filled with rapids of uncertainty and surprises around the bends, but also had beauty. I decided to look for beauty every day as I journeyed with cancer. Using my phone, I made a practice of taking photos of beautiful things I saw every day on my walks and often shared what I saw on social media, whether it was the beauty of a flowering cactus in Arizona, the details of a pine cone, patterns of leaves, a beautiful sunset, or a simple flower. By having my eyes focused on the beauty around me, I nurtured my own well-being and immersed myself in gratitude. By sharing the images with others, I encouraged them to appreciate the beauty around them.

Her cancer diagnosis also made Mary Sue clarify that she wanted to live closer to family, and she and her husband moved from Arizona to the mountains of Hood River, Oregon, near a white-water river lined with beautiful trees, alongside which she loves to walk. The beautiful scene she envisioned during her cancer treatment is very similar to the place she now calls home—a perfect example of a Connectedness experience.

Cancer Considerations

Share your thoughts
You generally trust what is happening without trying to make factual sense of it all. If you have a rare type of cancer, a surprising diagnosis, or a cancer where the cause is unknown, your Connectedness talents may help you accept this lack of causation more easily than others. Reflect on previous experiences and examine how you successfully approached these complex, unchartered life events. Work to articulate your thoughts and feelings with others about how you navigate things that are uncertain. You can create a tremendous ripple effect through your connections with others, which is why sharing your thoughts is so important.

Enjoy nature
Many times, people with the strength of Connectedness enjoy nature and the outdoors. If that sounds like you, look for ways to feed that enjoyment. Take walks or hikes, spend time gardening or growing flowers, ride your bike, or simply sit outside and enjoy the fresh air when that is all your energy will allow. If being in nature strongly resonates with you, make sure the spaces where you spend your time reflect that as well. This could be as simple as putting a plant on your desk in the office, opening your windows while you drive to the grocery store, or displaying a photo from an outdoor adventure to give you a visual reminder of your positive connection with nature.

Be a bridge-builder
You are likely comfortable with different groups, cultures, and thoughts outside of your own. This may motivate you to reach out to other cancer

survivors or cancer-related organizations. If you get a sense that you'd like to participate in the cancer world, beyond your role as patient and survivor, pay attention to what sparks your interests or passions. You may be drawn toward mentoring other cancer survivors, serving as a patient advocate, or getting involved in policy work and advocacy efforts. Consider how you can best contribute to your local, national, or global cancer communities.

On Gallup's *Theme Thursday* podcast, Mary Sue Ingraham shared how people with Connectedness are troubled by division but can be bridge builders by doing something with the connections they observe. She added, "Think globally, act locally. Find some way to build bridges where you can, with what you have, where you are."[33]

Listen closely to understand better

You may be a very good listener, which is helpful as you navigate medical decisions. Your listening skills will be beneficial as you reach out and connect with other cancer survivors to learn about their experiences. You may hear differing opinions and varied advice, so keep in mind that not all insight needs to be applied to your cancer experience. Keep tuning in to your listening skills and use the information you're gathering to create better questions. This practice of listening intently, noting the connections across a variety of sources, and asking even more questions will help you narrow in on the best treatment and healing plan moving forward for you.

Cancer Cautions

Reassure your supporters

Your supporters may have more of a need than you do to uncover the cause of your cancer or to have a definitive prognosis for you. If you experience uncommon side effects or surprising results from a procedure or treatment, they may have a lot more questions than you. If this is frustrating and

---

[33] Gallup CliftonStrengths. "Connectedness: Learning to Love All 34 Talent Themes." Available at: https://www.gallup.com/cliftonstrengths/en/251171/connectedness-learning-love-talent-themes.aspx.

draining, let them know that their anxious energy is not helping. Comfort them by explaining that you don't need to have all the answers. It may be as simple as "I understand it can be frustrating to have questions without answers. At this time, we just don't know and I'm okay with that."

Balance your intuition with data
Continue to check in with your intuition throughout your cancer experience. While relying on that strength of yours, be sure you are also considering the data and research being shared with you by your care team.

Consistency

People exceptionally talented in the Consistency theme are keenly aware of the need to treat people the same. They crave stable routines and clear rules and procedures that everyone can follow.

> The way to find your way through difficulty is not to find your way out, but to find your way up.
>
> —Karen Walrond, The Lightmaker's Manifesto

Fairness, balance, and predictability are important to you. You are keenly aware of the need to treat all people the same. When someone misses out on opportunities because of circumstances they can't control—or if they have an unfair advantage because of their connections or their background—this truly offends you. You are a guardian against inequity and favoritism. You believe that people function best in a consistent environment with clear rules that apply to everyone equally. These routines and rules comfort you because they support your need for fairness and predictability—and give each person the same chance to participate and show their worth.

Characteristics of Those with Consistency Talents

Fair	Leveling	Predictable
Just	Efficient	Equal
Compliant	Consistent	Practical

Cancer Connection

A cancer diagnosis would throw anyone for a loop, and there's not a strength that makes receiving this news any easier. People with Consistency as a strength tend to value balance and steadiness, and unfortunately, cancer usually doesn't honor these preferences. Given your knack for creating routines and establishing equilibrium, trust that you will naturally be able to steer this life disruption toward center. Your practical, objective approach to life and its challenges has served you well. Tap into previous times when you navigated difficult situations and identify what helped you work your way through these seasons of uncertainty.

You will establish your new normal and preferred method for approaching cancer. Take comfort in knowing you are a natural at creating structures, processes, and routines that guide your life. Use your skills in this new frontier as a patient and cancer survivor. Your care team will love your reliable approach with your adherence to the rules, medication compliance, and following their expectations and recommendations. They will consider you an ideal cancer patient.

Your principled approach to life will shape your cancer mindset and the thoughts and behaviors that are most helpful for you in navigating the phases of your treatment path. You are more likely to understand that not all diagnoses, treatment plans, and outcomes are equal or even fair as equality is one of your guideposts. Your approach to this cancer journey will calm your supporters who may be freaking out about your diagnosis. Continuing to demonstrate your Consistency strength will reassure your support team as they have historically regarded you as stable, steady, and a rock.

Cancer Considerations

Audit your habits
What habits do you already rely on that make you feel strong and energized? Consider your morning routine, commute, typical meals, exercise, hobbies, mindfulness or spiritual practices, and time spent with friends and family. Take an audit of these habits to evaluate which can effortlessly remain in place, which may need to be tweaked, and which need to be shelved for the time being.

Review your routines
As you evaluate your habits, consider new components in your life including appointments, treatments, fatigue, side effects, and energy levels. Work to maintain as many of your routines as possible through your diagnosis, treatment, and survivorship stages. Keep your list of routines nearby so that as you progress through treatment you can revise your standing list.

For example, you may have always started your day with a 60-minute walk outside before breakfast. As your treatment progresses and fatigue sets in, you may adjust this to a 30-minute walk. A few weeks after completing chemotherapy, you notice that your fatigue levels have decreased, so you bump your morning walk up to 45 minutes. As your strength improves and you reach your 60-minute walk, you will feel a sense of accomplishment and order being restored.

Keep a log of the impact of your treatment
To stick with as many of your previous routines and new cancer-impacted routines, pay close attention to the impact of treatment on your energy, appetite, mood, and sleep patterns. Typical advice for cancer patients is to write down these patterns and feelings to keep a log of what to expect in various time increments after treatment.

For example, track how you feel and what you notice 12 hours, 24 hours, two days, and five days after each treatment. This is an example of advice that is given to all cancer patients; however, it is much more likely to land for someone like you who is naturally structured and a creature of habit. If you notice that you feel normal for the first 48 hours after chemotherapy infusions, plan your work and personal schedule accordingly. This level of planning will help you manage your uncertainty. You may anticipate Days Three to Nine being more fatigue-filled and then you slowly rebuild your energy levels in Days 10 to 13, before heading back to the infusion chair for more chemo on Day 14.

One survivor shared that she liked knowing how the cycles would work so she could plan how to structure life around the side effects. Knowledge of the flow of your energy levels is critical to creating a pattern of work, play, and rest that is most appropriate for your life. This is something you know how to do naturally.

Look for ways to achieve efficiency and predictability
In the early days and weeks of your medical appointments, pay close attention to details and processes. Take note of things as small as where you park and check in, waiting room amenities, and various wait times. Are there things within your control that can help you feel more prepared for subsequent appointments? Do you like to be driven to appointments or do the driving? If you're at a large medical center, do you prefer to be dropped at the door or make the longer walk from the parking garage? Could you do anything to make the check-in process quicker or smoother? You're a big fan of predictable and efficient schedules, so do what you can to help make a smooth impact on your medical schedules, where possible.

Angie, a breast cancer survivor, noticed that she liked going to treatment on the same day at the same time with the same people. Thursdays became her treatment days, and she always took her husband and the same four friends along with her to appointments. Some people might get bored with the same cadence month after month, but for someone with Consistency talents, this approach helps create stability in a time full of uncertainty.

Prepare, note, and adjust

Depending on your care plan, you may experience repetitive procedures such as chemotherapy, radiation, physical therapy, and others. Although you may not be able to control the exact start times, your assigned chair or room, the medical professional administering treatment, or the length of your appointment, take note of the things you can impact. Your first of these experiences may naturally come with stress, anxiety, worry, and fear. No matter how much you read or how much advice you receive from other cancer survivors, it is still your first time and your unique experience. For my first chemo appointment, we had enough food, magazines, and blankets for an entire girl's week. We came fully prepared for the long end of the time estimate and then some. Of course, once I had completed round one and we understood the four-hour estimate was more likely than eight to ten, we adjusted our packing accordingly and never again wheeled a cooler into the infusion center.

Ask for support in your need for consistency

Once you have a treatment or two under your belt, what do you notice? What can you or your caretaker do to make these experiences feel more predictable? You may prefer reading in the waiting room and chatting during chemotherapy infusions rather than sleeping. If you have a favorite chair or nurse administering chemo, request what you prefer. Even if you can't have it, you will feel more in control asking. Anticipate trial and error with these processes but do take note of things you like and don't like along the way as it will help you create more of your ideal treatment arrangement.

Define your needs and set boundaries

What is your Cancer Nonnegotiable? Who needs to know your boundaries and guidelines? If a daily walk outside is a highlight of your day, make sure you set aside time for it. If having visitors stop by in the evening drains you, reserve visitors for when it supports you and ask your caretaker to help enforce this boundary. If you need consistency and predictability, you can have it.

Help your supporters understand what works for you

Given your value of fairness, you may not want extra attention or special treatment just because you have cancer. You realize this disease impacts millions of people and your mindset may be "Why not me?" Be prepared for people reaching out to you or your loved ones to see how they can provide support. They may offer to create a meal train to organize a schedule of dinners for your family, host a fundraiser golf outing to cover your travel and hotel expenses, or design custom rubber wristbands as a visual reminder of their support. If these or other examples feel uncomfortable to you, is there something else you'd appreciate? You may prefer smaller, less visible gestures such as people joining you on your morning walk, taking your children to a movie, or gift cards you can easily put toward dinner on nights when you're too tired to cook. Steering your supporters in the right direction is different from being stubborn and ungrateful. They truly want to help, and honoring your unique wishes creates a win-win for everyone.

Make backup plans to tackle inconsistency

Audit your time—where are you spending it and what commitments may need to be modified or removed from your schedule during treatment? You will feel efficient and in control of your schedule by conducting this audit in advance rather than a day-by-day, flexible approach. For example, you may decide to cut back on your volunteering activities. Let's say you're involved in filling bags at the local food bank, serving on the Boys & Girls Club board, and coaching your kids' soccer team. You may decide to limit these outside service activities to account for your fatigue. But you notice that the idea of giving up coaching makes you angry and sad. If you're still able to commit the time and energy to coaching, give it a go, but make sure to have backup plans in place for days when your medical treatments interfere, or your fatigue makes it too difficult. These backup plans will reduce your stress because you hate inconsistency and unpredictability.

Use your strength for fairness

As a person with a natural eye for fairness and equality, do you notice anything that seems unfair in the world of cancer? This may take months or even years to notice given how large and overwhelming this space can be. Take note of what you're feeling if you find yourself upset by data, statistics, stories, or experiences. You may be struck by inequalities based on race, gender, age, economic class, location, or type of cancer. Consider joining a local support group, cancer organization, or advocacy network if you feel compelled to dig in, learn more, or act.

My husband and I have gotten involved with advocacy efforts through the American Cancer Society and the National Breast Cancer Coalition (NBCC). Our motivations may have been driven by our strengths as Consistency is high for him, and Belief is high for me. We are members of the American Cancer Society Cancer Action Network (ACS CAN) which views health equity as "everyone having a fair and just opportunity to prevent, find, treat, and survive cancer. It requires us to eliminate barriers and address needs to ensure everyone has the same opportunity to be healthy and cancer-free." And NBCC "combines the power of advocacy, education, policy and research to unite around one goal: ending breast cancer."[34] This involvement led us to travel to Washington, D.C., multiple times with a team of advocates from Iowa to meet with our legislators and encourage them to support ACS CAN's and NBCC's top priorities. Kent and I both learned a lot about health disparities through this education and advocacy work with ACS CAN and NBCC as well as our observations and reflections during my cancer treatment.

Cancer Cautions

Acknowledge that your cancer is specific

Because you believe in fairness and prize efficiency, be careful not to flatten the specifics of your diagnosis. You may have the same type of cancer

---

34 Breast Cancer Advocacy, National Breast Cancer Coalition: https://www.stopbreastcancer.org.

as somebody else, such as prostate or ovarian, but you may have variances in stage, grade, tumor size, genetic markers, or a variety of other factors that impact your treatment. Pay attention to the specifics of your cancer and don't lose sight of the treatment you need. Avoid reading or listening to information that is too general and keep an eye on thoughts you have like "If that was good enough for Malik, it's good enough for me." Be careful not to overgeneralize cancer types, treatments, or prognoses. It is critical to make sure you are receiving customized diagnosis and treatment information from an accredited institution and provider.

Identify your MO for dealing with change
Having a plan and a preferred MO (mode of operating) is a great approach for you. Keep in mind that it may be more of a draft or an outline. You can only control what you can control and will need to channel some patience and flexibility through this process, which can be challenging since you prefer standards and predictability. It's helpful to understand what tactics or what people have helped you with adapting to changing circumstances in the past. Leverage those strategies or people to help you through what will undoubtedly be more of a road under construction with twists and turns than a smooth racetrack with calculated pit stops.

Expect varied outcomes and avoid comparisons
Despite the incredible medical advances in cancer treatment, the disease still significantly impacts the lives it touches. You may have the exact same procedure as another cancer survivor yet experience different results and outcomes. Two surgeries may be technically the same; however, two patients experience different recovery times and side effects. It is natural to play the comparison game when you value fairness, so keep in mind the possibility of varied outcomes. It can be especially overwhelming to question why outcomes vary between you and a family member, friend, or loved one if you have someone close to you who has experienced cancer. Given you are a person who values rules and fairness, this may lead you to experience a range of emotions including bitterness, resentment, and guilt. I've heard numerous cancer survivors share how hard it was to

lose a friend to the same type of cancer they had, and the experience left them asking, "Why me? Why are they gone and I'm still here?" Survivor's guilt is a real experience for many cancer survivors. If you encounter it, seek out a support group, fellow survivor, or therapist to process through those feelings.

Context

People exceptionally talented in the Context theme enjoy thinking about the past. They understand the present by researching its history.

You look back—because that is where the answers lie. You look to the past to make sense of the present. Faced with new people and new situations, it will take you a little time to orient yourself. Until you understand the history and underlying structure of something, you might see the present as an unstable, confusing clamor of competing voices. But when you look back, your mind sees original plans, initial intentions, and lessons learned. Knowing this history brings you confidence. You make better decisions because you know what has—and hasn't—worked in the past. You become a better partner because you appreciate how your colleagues became who they are. And counterintuitively, you become wiser about the future because you won't repeat the mistakes of the past.

You are incredibly talented in digging for the details, headlines, archives, and backstory. Embrace that uniqueness to uncover cancer-related background knowledge that will help to shape your path forward.

Characteristics of Those with Context Talents

Historical	Perceptive	Collecting
Orienting	Highlighting	Studious

Cancer Connection

You are naturally an inquisitive, curious, and thoughtful person. You may have lots of questions surrounding your diagnosis revolving around "How did we get here?" For many of us, receiving a cancer diagnosis is a shock to our system and rocks our world. While many cancer survivors also have a lot of questions, you are incredibly talented in digging for the details, headlines, archives, and backstory. Embrace that uniqueness as you work to uncover cancer-related background knowledge that will help to shape your path forward.

If this is an unexpected diagnosis for you, be patient with yourself as you adjust to your new current state. You prefer to understand the present through the lens of the past. You like to see the breadcrumb trail and how one thing led to the next. In the case of many cancer diagnoses, your medical team may not be able to pinpoint exactly why or how you developed the disease. Be prepared to make medical decisions and take steps forward without the ability to trace your footsteps entirely back to the root cause.

As you navigate your cancer experience, embrace your need for context. Ask detailed questions of your care team, and allow yourself time to pause, reflect, and think about what else you need to know. Your mindset, energy levels, and decisions will be better after you have had sufficient time to review, reflect, and research your options. The time you allow yourself to digest and examine the final blueprint for your care will increase your level of confidence in the steps moving forward.

Cancer Considerations

Seek the context you need

You will be more comfortable proceeding through your treatment and recovery once you understand the past and what brought you to this current state with your health as much as you can. Help your medical team and loved ones understand this natural inclination of yours. What could be perceived as resistance or denial is a prerequisite for you to move forward with confidence.

Depending on the temperaments and talents of your medical team and support system, you may feel rushed, pressured, and annoyed because of when they need you to make decisions or start your treatment. If that happens, it may be helpful to explain to them "I need time to process and think. I need more context on this diagnosis, the treatment options, and examples of what has worked well for other cancer survivors to move forward. Please be patient with me."

There may be circumstances where a timely decision is required, such as to secure an in-demand surgeon or begin treating an aggressive form of cancer immediately. In those situations, tell your care team members and loved ones that you may need more of their help processing information to make a timely decision and not slow down your treatment.

Talk with people who have been on the same path

Talk with others who have gone through a similar cancer experience. Ask them reflective and contextual questions:
- What were the most helpful tools or resources for you?
- What did you learn along the way?
- Looking back, what do you know now that you wish you knew then?
- What would you do differently?

Their stories will provide insight and background to help inform your path ahead. You may intentionally try to recreate the strategies that were helpful for them. It may calm you to remember that millions of people faced cancer before you, and you'll be able to face it too.

Seek out long-term cancer survivors who experienced a cancer diagnosis 10–20 years ago for wisdom. Their stories and advice will give you hope and perspective. If they no longer show evidence of disease and their cancer follow-ups are few to none, they will have a unique rearview mirror–type perspective. Long-term survivors living with Stage 4 cancer will have a long-range lens, in addition to a close-up zoom lens if they are actively engaged in treatment and medical appointments. These people may very well become your cancer mentors as their insights and advice from the past and present will help you through your cancer experience.

I vividly remember talking with a friend's mother two months into my cancer diagnosis during the most difficult stretch of my chemotherapy. At that point, Kathy was a 20-year breast cancer and lung cancer survivor. She is naturally caring and empathetic and asked me how I was doing with everything. I told her I recently learned that breast cancer commonly recurs and feared going through all of this only to get sick again. She said she remembered feeling that way and I asked, for how long? Without hesitation, she replied, "About five years." It was a straightforward conversation and one I reflected on countless times during the five years following my diagnosis. When fear and anxiety about the unknown future snuck up on me, I calmly put myself back in that kitchen with Kathy to remember that my worry was common and would gradually lessen.

Understand your family history
Dig deep into your family medical history and genetic predispositions, if this information is available. This is often a recommendation for cancer patients; however, it will just be another task on their cancer to-do list. For you, you may feel energized to learn the health histories available for your grandparents, parents, aunts, uncles, and siblings. Are there any clues from your biological relatives that could help you and your medical team better understand your current health situation? This may be difficult if you were adopted, family members have passed away, or information was not properly recorded. Do what you can to use your strength of Context to orient yourself.

Remember past successes
You may be blessed with a better memory than most. Challenge yourself to reflect on your past successes in navigating adversity, obstacles, or challenges. Reflect on these questions:
- What was the obstacle or challenge?
- What successful actions did you take to overcome this adversity?
- What helped you mentally, physically, or emotionally?
- What people, tools, resources, or strategies were beneficial?

After you've spent time thinking about your history with adversity, are there any things you did or didn't do that are applicable to your cancer journey? How can you repeat these successful approaches and make the most of the lessons you've learned from previous challenges? Perhaps you've experienced the loss of a loved one and struggled with grief. If you felt best on the days you exercised in the morning and spent quality time with a close friend over coffee or lunch, that lesson may transfer well into your new cancer path. Or maybe you struggled with relocation to a new city or the end of a romantic relationship. As you reflect on those experiences, you may realize that meeting new people through your spiritual community helped you navigate those changes. Spend more time digging into what helped, rather than hurt, during previous hardships and you will find this reflection time valuable and encouraging.

Get to know your care team
Use your Context talents to build relationships with your care team and supporters. You may feel stronger by hearing personal stories of your care team. Ask about where they are from, what they studied, and how their medical career has progressed. Ask them about the best outcomes their patients have experienced and what they think you can apply from those patients' experiences to your cancer. It will energize you to learn the backstory of your team, and it will energize them to feel your genuine interest in past successes.

Reflect on the history of cancer and acknowledge advancements
People with Context as a strength tend to value history and the past. Do you happen to be curious about the history of cancer as a disease or your specific type of cancer? If so, your Context strength can help you dig deep into this curiosity. Ask your oncologist about the history of your kind of cancer and how treatment has changed over the decades. Ask how much progress has been made on disease prevention, diagnosis, treatment, or survival. Follow your need to look back as a way to draw on this strength.

You may be somebody who enjoys reading, and this could be a very valuable source of energy for you. If you really want to dig in, check out *The Emperor of All Maladies: A Biography of Cancer* written by cancer physician, researcher, and Pulitzer Prize–winning author Siddhartha Mukherjee.[35] While Context is not high on my list of strengths, I did listen to the 22-hour book on Audible and was fascinated to learn more about the complexity of the disease and the stories of people such as Dr. Sidney Farber, known as the father of modern chemotherapy, who was involved in bringing the cancer conversation to the forefront.[36] His brother Darwin shared, "He was a medical diplomat. He saw that if cancer was going to be conquered, it would require a concerted effort and major funding commitment by Congress." According to the Dana–Farber Institute, he was a star presenter at congressional hearings and his persuasive advocacy played a significant role in nearly quadrupling the annual budget in the fifties and sixties of the National Cancer Institute. If a historical perspective of cancer is intriguing to you, *The Emperor of All Maladies* book, or the 2015 six-hour film written and produced by Ken Burns, might be right up your alley.

Given your preference for thinking about the past, take a moment to give this some consideration. If you had to be diagnosed with this disease, outcomes are better now than 10, 20, or 30 years ago. This is

---

35   Mukherjee, Siddhartha (2010). *The Emperor of All Maladies: A Biography of Cancer.* Scribner.

36   Dana–Farber Cancer Institute (undated). "Sidney Farber, MD: A Career in Cancer Research Driven by the Power of an Idea." Available at: https://www.dana-farber.org/about/history/sidney-farber.

not to make light of your diagnosis, but to encourage you to acknowledge the research, technology, medications, clinical trials, and overall advancements that have been made or improved over the last 40 years. The last two sentences aren't cruel attempts to show you a silver lining or to encourage gratitude. They are based on multiple experiences I've had as a cancer survivor.

After my double mastectomy in 2017, my pathology results returned that I had pCR or pathologic complete response. This was the best possible outcome for us and one that only 10% of people with my type of tumors receive. It was absolutely incredible news, and I could hear it in the voices of my oncologist and surgeon when they called with the results. The next step for me was to take a daily pill for five years called tamoxifen, a hormone therapy drug that greatly reduces the chance of recurrence. The option of radiation was less clear, given the pCR results. There was a clinical trial underway to understand if radiation helped improve survival rates and reduce recurrence for patients who received pCR. However, at the time I had to make this decision, that data was unavailable. I remember venting to my surgeon saying, "It's just frustrating to have so many unknowns." I'll never forget her calmly talking me through the situation and sharing, "Actually, we do know a lot about breast cancer. We know so much more now than we did 20 years ago." In that moment, Dr. Sugg's nod to the history of cancer reassured me of my situation and that I was sitting in as good a position as possible.

Seven years later, I underwent a delayed breast reconstruction surgery called DIEP flap.[37] According to the medical practice PRMA in San Antonio where I received treatment, "The DIEP flap is the most advanced form of breast reconstruction available today. It uses the patient's own abdominal tissue to restore a natural, warm, soft breast after mastectomy." When I weighed my surgery options in 2017, I didn't know anyone who had opted for DIEP flap. Now, I personally know over 50 women who have been diagnosed with breast cancer, yet still only five

---

37 DIEP Flap Breast Reconstruction for Natural Breasts: https://prma-enhance.com/breast-reconstruction/diep-flap.

who have opted for that surgery. It is becoming increasingly prevalent, a testament to medical advancements. If my mother had been diagnosed with breast cancer at the age of 39 like me, the DIEP flap surgery option wouldn't have been available.

Additionally, I've met multiple people who have benefited from the drug Herceptin, which was approved by the Federal Drug Administration (FDA) to treat HER2+ early stage breast cancer in 2006. One survivor I interviewed is clear to point out, "Herceptin was and still is a game changer for me and so many people that has allowed us to survive and thrive past this horrible disease." While there is still much work to be done, there have been tremendous advances in medical innovation and cancer research. Use this strength to learn about your type of cancer and how treatment has evolved.

Learn how others have walked with cancer

You also may find it helpful to read biographies and memoirs about other cancer survivors. For example, if you are fascinated by history, read about famous journalists or political figures who have endured cancer. If you are a sports fan, read books or articles about famous athletes and coaches who have battled cancer. If illness or fatigue prevents you from reading, consider seeking out audiobooks, podcasts, or movies. You may be energized by reading, hearing, or seeing others' stories of their walks with cancer.

Keep a record of your experience

Are there any cancer memories, souvenirs, or memorabilia that you'd like to keep? Since you enjoy looking back at the past, you may enjoy reflecting on this experience in the future. Consider capturing memories in a journal. If you enjoy writing, treat yourself to a nice notebook or place to record your thoughts. Photographs and videos are always powerful mementos of the past. Many cancer survivors share photos with a select group of friends and family, or to the broader public online if that feels comfortable. These visual representations can serve as powerful reminders for all that you faced and how far you've come as you look back months and hopefully years down the road.

Compare your earlier experience
If you have progressed beyond active treatment and are returning for follow-up visits, reexperience the feelings you had as you were actively engaged in your treatment. Try to remember what your energy levels were at that time compared to now. Reflect on your previous physical and emotional states in waiting rooms and doctor's offices. You may have felt all kinds of things such as exhausted, nauseated, achy, impatient, bald, worried, scared, or depressed. You likely feel much better now than during your most tiring days of blood draws, chemotherapy, surgeries, radiation, or physical therapy. Although your health may not be fully restored to before your diagnosis, this reflective perspective will give you a boost and a reminder of your strength, perseverance, and resiliency.

Unearth the history of healthcare
If you're interested in political advocacy, you may be fascinated by the history of healthcare decisions in your district, state, or country. Having knowledge of past decisions and efforts can be invaluable when working to influence elected officials.

Cancer Cautions

Focus on outcomes, not blame
Although you are likely going to want to understand how or why you have cancer, be careful not to dwell on this for long. It can be maddening to focus on the variety of potential causes of your disease. Work to make sure your desire to understand what led to this diagnosis is productive, reasonable, and helpful for future outcomes you're trying to achieve. Don't beat yourself up by digging into causes such as food, diet, or beauty product ingredients. You're here. You have cancer. In other words, don't let this strength pull you into rumination or self blame.

Curate your resources, judiciously

You are a great historian and collector of memories. Just remember that you don't have to keep everything you've collected. In the early days of your diagnosis, every brochure and xeroxed copy of information may feel like gold to you as you're desperate for answers and context. As you progress through your diagnosis, treatment, and further stages, the information or memories you initially collected may weigh you down. Make it a practice to cull your resources—both physical and electronic—and reduce your load.

Call for support as you need

Making decisions by using the past to be informed is one of your great strengths. If you find yourself stuck spending too much time researching or trying to understand the past, reach out for help. Share your challenge with your medical team, caregiver, or spiritual and social supporters. Look for people who help ground you in the present as well as those visionaries who inspire you with ideas about the future. Consider asking for a referral to a psychologist, mental health therapist, or support group to help you stay present and looking forward to your future.

Deliberative

People exceptionally talented in the Deliberative theme are best described by the serious care they take in making decisions. They anticipate risks and move forward cautiously.

You are a careful and vigilant person who approaches life with a certain reserve. You know that the world is an unpredictable place. Even when everything seems in order, beneath the surface, you sense many risks. Rather than ignoring these risks, you identify, assess, and reduce each one. You like to plan ahead so you can anticipate what might go wrong. You select your friends cautiously and keep your opinions to yourself about personal matters. You are careful not to give too much praise and recognition. For you, life is not a popularity contest. While you might think others make decisions quickly and recklessly, you trust your naturally good judgment. You identify dangers, weigh their impact, and move forward carefully.

My Deliberative strength helped me to be forward-thinking and to prevent problems. Listen to this strength of yours.

—Chris, melanoma survivor

Characteristics of Those with Deliberative Talents

Careful	Conservative	Thoughtful	Confidential
Vigilant	Private	Guarded	Sensible
Serious	Observant	Risk-averse	Compliant

Cancer Connection

Your careful and thoughtful approach to life will be beneficial as you navigate your cancer experience. There are a lot of decisions to make along the way, from where you pursue medical care to the type of treatment you select to the changes you make to your daily schedule. You take your time when making big decisions, anticipate what could go wrong, and have a plan for the different scenarios.

You probably don't like to be rushed into making decisions, so make sure to share that preference with the people around you who are impacted by your diagnosis too. Your diagnosis may create an energy in others that feels like anxiousness, intensity, and eagerness to move forward. If you'd like, share with them that you understand this is serious and you also want to proceed with care. Tell them that you want to be confident in your decisions, and that your confidence usually increases with a little extra time to reflect. The expression "Slow and steady wins the race," from Aesop's fable "The Tortoise and the Hare" may be fitting for how you make decisions. In most cases—not all—taking a few extra days or sometimes weeks will not greatly affect your course of treatment or the options available to you. Ask your potential care team about the ideal timeframe for you to make treatment decisions and plan accordingly.

There are certainly obstacles that go hand in hand with a cancer diagnosis. These can range from side effects of treatment like nausea and fatigue to adjusting your work schedule to managing the costs involved in gas, meals, and overnight stays for medical care. You are less likely than others to feel down or defeated when faced with these challenges if you have time to anticipate and plan for them in advance. Reassure others that you are not a pessimist or a downer, but that your Deliberative strength helps you see risk clearly, and often before most people. Let them know that thinking through the different paths, possibilities, and potential problems is helpful for you in making your best decisions and plans. Chris is a Stage 3 melanoma cancer survivor with the Deliberative strength and shared that it "helped me be forward-thinking and to prevent problems. Listen to this strength of yours."

Cancer Considerations

You are comfortable evaluating your options
You will evaluate all your options in a thoughtful, controlled manner. Many cancer survivors default to the most common or safest option without much additional thought. Your willingness to be patient may open up more possibilities for your treatment options. You may explore multiple health centers, oncologists, or surgical approaches before making major decisions. This approach involves additional time on the front end, but it is time you are willing to spend if it could improve your health outcomes. Even if after evaluating multiple options, you still land on the most selected path, you will feel confident in that decision due to the additional time you committed to the process.

Plan B's come naturally
You are probably used to thinking through potential challenges, making backup plans, and creating a Plan B. This can be a definite advantage as you move through the phases of your cancer treatment. It is common for cancer surgeons to share their going in approach and their backup plan. For example, you may go into surgery for a mastectomy without knowing if they will remove a small number of lymph nodes under your armpit area or a much larger number through a procedure called an axillary lymph node dissection. This procedure increases your risk of lymphedema, or swelling in your arm, due to a buildup of lymph fluid. It is

stressful going into a major surgery not knowing which path your surgeon will select. Your natural way of processing big decisions will prepare you for this type of situation since you are accustomed to considering at least two paths for every challenge you face.

Identify past decision-making partners
When faced with big decisions in your life, who helps you weigh your options and gain the momentum you need to move forward? Think of choices you've had in the past whether they were related to your career, a relationship, a significant purchase, or a medical procedure. Was there a certain person or group of people you turned to or did you usually rely on an expert in that arena?

Explore how others face similar decisions
You may benefit from hearing how other people process the pros, cons, considerations, and risks of your medical decisions. You may not take the same approach or make the same decision as these people, but hearing their perspectives can be a valuable process.

Ask if caution is valuable
You are naturally cautious and may take the conservative route in most of your decisions. Before proceeding with medical decisions, ask yourself, "Is now the time where being cautious is valuable?" It very well may be, but it's worth pausing to ask the question. If you aren't sure of the answer, ask your care team and trusted supporters for their insight. You may not select a riskier surgery or medication in the long run, but at least you will have considered it as you weighed your options.

Do you want sight of the agenda?
You tend to be a private person and prefer to think before you talk. This preference may influence your medical appointments and how you approach sharing your health updates. People with the Deliberative strength often say that they do better in meetings if they see an agenda in advance. Is it possible for you to ask your oncologist or other care providers, "What can

I expect for our next appointment?" Understanding the plan for the next visit will help you prepare for that moment in advance.

Take someone with you to appointments
During appointments, do your best to ensure that your caregiver or somebody closely involved with your treatment plan attends. If you receive information and need time to process, turn to this trusted person and say, "What questions do you have about this information?" or "What do you think I need to consider?" Hearing their questions and thoughts will buy you additional time to process the information from your oncologist, surgeon, or other provider. You may need that time to soak in the information and think of questions to ask. Additionally, you can always ask for time to think and explain that it helps you make your best decisions.

It's okay not to share everything
While some cancer survivors share their diagnoses and health updates with hundreds or even thousands of people on social media, you may prefer to keep your health information contained to a much smaller circle. Honor this instinctual feeling of yours and remind yourself to share when you are comfortable.

With your preference of thinking, set yourself up to have time to respond to questions or inquiries from people who care about you. For example, a trusted friend or family member provides occasional updates to a small group instead of you sending emails or texts. This creates space and reduces the overwhelming and bombarding feeling of you receiving questions and responses instantly.

Cancer Cautions

You don't have to make big decisions alone
Check in with yourself and your medical team about the length of time you have before they recommend you decide on a course of treatment. You put great thought and care into making difficult decisions, and this

has always served you well. Reach out for additional help if you find yourself hesitating, overwhelmed, or unable to move forward. This help may come from your medical team, a therapist, or a trusted friend or family member. Do not let fear lead you to delay a decision if time will critically impact your options and health outcomes.

Seek a balanced view

While you innately see bumps in the road before the rest of us, make sure you aren't creating potholes in your mind if the pavement is mostly smooth. Most medical treatments, procedures, and medications come with some level of risk. Do not confuse risk with danger. If you find yourself dwelling on the risk, check in with your care team for more information, data, and statistics before putting too much weight on your fears and potential worse case scenarios.

Developer

People exceptionally talented in the Developer theme recognize and cultivate the potential in others. They spot the signs of each small improvement and love when they see someone make progress.

You see potential in people, and this draws you to them. In your view, no individual is fully formed. On the contrary, each person is a work in progress and full of possibilities. You want other people to succeed, so you look for ways to challenge them and help them grow. And all the while, you are on the lookout for signs of growth in others—a slight improvement in a skill, a behavior learned or modified, a glimpse of excellence. For you, these small increments—invisible to some—are proof of someone beginning to realize their potential. These signs of growth in others are your fuel. They bring you strength and satisfaction. Others will come to you for help and encouragement—not only because you have Developer talent, but because they know that helping others is genuinely fulfilling for you.

People are like stained-glass windows. They sparkle and shine when the sun is out, but when the darkness sets in, their true beauty is revealed only if there is a light from within.

—Elisabeth Kübler-Ross, creator of the five stages of grief

Characteristics of Those with Developer Talents

Patient	Effective	Inventing
Observant	Self-sacrificing	Perceptive
Encouraging	Others-oriented	Growth-oriented
Helpful		

Cancer Connection

If each strength were just one picture, Developer would be a seed sprouting into a beautiful flower. You come alive when you see people grow. You love to be a part of that process by sharing your insights, expertise, encouragement, and praise. As you face your cancer diagnosis, continue to share your love of progress with the people you encounter. You may notice the person at the registration desk handling multiple phone calls, answering questions from coworkers, and organizing paperwork and hospital wristbands. Share what you notice about the way they are shifting gears, staying calm, and delivering friendly patient care. They will probably look at you like you told them they won the lottery since many people do not receive enough positive recognition at their workplace. This shared connection as you display your supportive disposition with your care team will boost your energy levels along the way.

You have likely always looked for ways to help other people, whether that's training a new bank teller how to make a deposit, encouraging the nervous new waiter memorizing your dinner order, or teaching your niece how to tie her shoelaces. You get a kick out of watching people try new things and get better with each attempt. Could you turn that cheering section toward yourself while you learn something new, like how to play the piano, plant a small pot of herbs, or cook a healthy new recipe? If there is an area in your life where you would like to learn something new or expand on your current ability level, now might be a good time to take small steps in that area as it will keep your spirits up during treatment.

As you progress through your cancer experience, take note of people, activities, or organizations you are drawn to support. Pay attention if there are certain things you learn about healthcare or cancer that you want to share with others. You don't have to act on these insights now, but they may be signs of how you can share your strength in the future. You may enjoy mentoring a newly diagnosed cancer survivor, teaching others yoga, or serving as a patient advocate to help improve training processes within the hospital. Your drive for progress is typically outward focused but do your best to take note of how you are blossoming and growing during this challenging experience as well. What you see will likely amaze you.

Cancer Considerations

You are a natural teacher
Is there anyone you think would like to learn more about your cancer experience? Developer is high on my list of strengths, and I enjoyed having my friends and family join me at chemotherapy appointments. I thought it was fun to share specifics about how the process works, such as the fact they weigh you and draw labs before treatment. This ensures that your blood counts are at a level conducive to receiving chemo and your weight is used to know exactly how much chemotherapy to administer. I thought that was pretty cool, and I found myself smiling and gaining energy when I had a chance to share this interesting information with others.

Look for opportunities for mutual encouragement
While you are going through your cancer experience, is there anyone you can encourage along the way? Early in my diagnosis, I was introduced to another breast cancer survivor, Laurel. We were the same age, both had two young children, shared the same oncologist, and our chemo appointments landed on the same day. I found comfort in going through treatment with another person, and we both offered encouragement to each other. We have remained friends over eight years after our first introduction in the infusion center.

Likewise, is there a cancer survivor you can connect with who is a few weeks ahead of you in the treatment cycle? You are good at seeing potential and what can be, and it will be helpful for you to talk with somebody who is a few steps ahead in the process.

Mentor someone newly diagnosed
As you continue gaining weeks, months, and years of experience as a cancer survivor, you will likely be introduced to people who are newly diagnosed. Although you never want anyone else to experience cancer, you will also realize that survivors can give each other unique support. When we encourage each other, it's like there's an extra shot of espresso in your latte. One cancer survivor, Donna, shared that she has helped mentor at least 15 people through the early parts of their diagnosis. Developer is one of Donna's top strengths so providing this guidance is instinctive and rewarding for her.

If your fatigue won't allow it, no problem. Tuck this consideration away for when you have more energy to support another person, whether that's through their cancer diagnosis or a completely different challenge.

Celebrate the small wins
Look to incorporate things to celebrate into your cancer experience. Many people with the Developer strength say they enjoy celebrating the small wins just as much as the big milestones, like ringing the bell after finishing chemo or radiation. Feeling less nauseated than last week and able to drive your kids to school every day this week? That's a win. Eyelashes and eyebrows sticking around through one more treatment? Check! Evaluate the progress you make each week and take comfort in each of these small victories.

Cancer Cautions

Challenge your tendency to show patience
Are you spending too much time waiting on something that is only showing slight signs of improvement? For example, you may have significant

side effects on your fingernails and toenails due to chemotherapy. Chemo damages things that grow fast, like tumors, but it can also cause damage to peripheral body parts that grow fast, like your hair and nails. It may be painful and unsightly, but you spot subtle improvements each day and decide to take a wait-and-see approach. This may be a time to reach out to experts, such as a dermatologist or podiatrist, sooner than later. Challenge yourself to ask, "Is this progress good enough or would faster be better for my health outcomes?" Your patience is certainly an admirable quality, but there are times when it's helpful to be a bit impatient when it comes to your health.

Reject poor performance

Are you taking it too easy on your medical providers? You tend to see potential in others, but make sure you aren't putting up with poor performance from your care team because you know they can improve. You don't need to wait around for them while they get better at their job.

Not everyone wants ongoing support

There may be some cancer survivors who do not want your continued support. Don't take this personally and think that you said or did something wrong. For example, your coworker may connect you with another survivor. You share helpful advice over the phone, they thank you for making the time to connect but then do not respond to a few follow-up texts. I had an experience like this where I helped somebody on the front end of their diagnosis and it was clear that one phone call from me was exactly what they needed and no more. I followed up with their close friend who connected us, and she validated that this cancer survivor was doing great and had all the support they needed for the next phases of their treatment plan. Remind yourself that people may need various levels of support and guidance depending on where they are in their treatment and healing process.

Discipline

People exceptionally talented in the Discipline theme enjoy routine and structure. Their world is best described by the order they create.

> I had a need to organize something. I had no control over so much of it, but organization gives me a sense of control and that there are things I can do to make my life and other people's lives easier.
>
> —Sharon (1947–2022), breast cancer survivor

Your life needs to be predictable, ordered, and planned. You instinctively impose structure on your world by setting up routines and focusing on timelines and deadlines. You break long-term projects into specific short-term plans, and you work through each plan diligently. You are not necessarily neat and clean, but you do crave precision. Faced with the messiness of life, you want to feel in control. Routines, timelines, and structure all help create that feeling of control. Your dislike of surprises, your impatience with errors, your routines and your attention to detail aren't controlling behaviors that limit you and others. Rather, they are your instinctive method for maintaining progress and productivity in the face of life's many distractions.

Characteristics of Those with Discipline Talents

Predictable	Organized	Meticulous	Neat
Timely	Planned	Detail-oriented	Efficient
Structured	Orderly	Rehearsed	Exact

Cancer Connection

Discipline is an extremely rare strength. At the time of this book's publication, it was one of the five rarest strengths, out of 34, in the world.[38] You are a rarity, and you can use this to make your cancer experience feel safer and more orderly. Cancer may feel threatening for many reasons, including throwing your sense of structure and efficiency into turmoil. What you want is to use your rare strength to your advantage to deal with the chaos and unpredictability that a cancer diagnosis often brings. Cancer is not easy for most people to manage, and it could prove extra challenging as you typically prefer structure and order—but it doesn't have to.

One of the best ways to use this strength is to relax into following any set regimens and treatment schedules that your cancer providers create. You will find comfort in the rhythm and flow of your treatment routines. Other survivors who prefer spontaneity and flexibility in their daily lives may struggle more with schedules, but you can conserve energy and use it to develop more flexibility when needed.

Since your life has taken this unexpected turn, consider what schedules or spaces need to be organized. As Traci prepares for her double mastectomy surgery, her husband and two college-aged children notice that her organization skills are kicking into high gear. She is buying a recliner to aid in her rest and recovery from surgery, but timing that purchase

---

38 Gallup CliftonStrengths, "Discipline: Learning to Love All 34 Talent Themes." Available at: https://www.gallup.com/cliftonstrengths/en/251144/discipline-learning-love-talent-themes.aspx.

to follow the installation of new carpet. She laughed when telling me, "My family is joking that I'm nesting. Preparing for this surgery and my downtime is similar, in a sense, because I know it's a busy time of year for my family and I just want the house to be in order." She instinctively knows that her recovery will feel smoother for everyone if those pieces are in place in advance of her surgery. Similarly, if you are a parent or caretaker of a loved one or pet, you may need assistance with supporting their lives. Take an inventory of all that potentially needs to be arranged, including any of the following:

- Medical supplies such prescriptions, medications, wigs, walkers, recliners, shower chairs, or other home health supplies
- Physical spaces where you're spending more time such as a home office, porch, couch, or bedroom
- Recurring appointments such as your annual checkup, dentist, eye, oil changes, or caring for your yard
- Work schedules, potentially considering reducing hours, taking days off, or requesting a leave of absence
- Communication with family and friends regarding your health status and updates, depending on the amount you are sharing and the breadth of who receives the updates
- Family and personal commitments, such as previously scheduled plans, activities, or trips

Cancer Considerations

You can do more with less

Curt Liesveld, Senior Consultant at Gallup and my Strengths teacher, beautifully described people with Discipline as "very good at managing limited personal resources by creating and following a plan. They bring order to chaos."[39] You have a knack for minimizing outside noise and

---

39 Gallup CliftonStrengths, "Discipline: Learning to Love All 34 Talent Themes." Available at: https://www.gallup.com/cliftonstrengths/en/251144/discipline-learning-love-talent-themes.aspx.

distractions. You can simplify things and do more with less, which you will be doing during your cancer treatment. Depending on your type of cancer and where you're at in your treatment plan, you may be navigating multiple kinds of *less* including:

- Energy
- Strength
- Appetite
- Hair
- Clothes that fit
- Calmness or clarity
- Financial resources
- Free time

One step at a time

You are a natural at breaking long-term goals into short-term steps. There are typically multiple phases and interventions in a cancer treatment plan. Your ability to break these down into doable steps will serve you well. Examples of phases and treatment types include screening and imaging, diagnosis, genetic testing, immunotherapy, surgery, chemotherapy, radiation, hormone therapy, and medication—of course, your treatment will be unique and may or may not include these tests and elements. Cancer phases and treatment may be broken into subcategories or include multiple sessions. Many cancer survivors track treatments numerically or by percentage, either mentally or by sharing updates with their supporters. People may share a photo with one hand in the air, fingers spread wide to indicate they have completed their fifth session in a series of radiation or chemotherapy treatments. Others have mentioned things like "I'm halfway there" or "I'm 75% finished with this part of the plan."

Plan the work and work the plan

I imagine you have detailed plans for anything from vacation itineraries to DIY home projects to family reunions. Your cancer diagnosis was not something you elected to have happen nor is it anything like a vacation, but it is still something that has many steps and milestones. Take your experience of managing projects or events and channel your considerable skills into planning and coordinating the tasks and steps involved in your cancer care.

The project plan you develop will support your need for preparedness, and you will be energized by the creation process as well. Barb is a friend, neighbor, and breast cancer survivor, and her job is in project management for a global organization. She shared, "I made lists of the supplies I needed for my upcoming surgery and what we needed at home during my recovery. I ordered drain pockets, a shower pouch, and arranged for groceries to be delivered during my downtime. I manage projects every day at work, so taking these steps during my cancer treatment helped me feel organized and prepared for what was ahead."

Depending on your prognosis, you may need to use your Discipline strength for advance care planning. This could include creating a living will, selecting a person to make medical decisions if you are unable, designating a power of attorney or somebody to assist in managing your finances, in-home care or hospice service preferences, and potentially communicating your last wishes to loved ones. Our neighbor and my breast cancer mentor, Sharon, survived metastatic breast cancer for 12 years. When I interviewed her about her Discipline strength just six months before she passed away, Sharon shared:

> As it relates to my cancer journey, I had a need to organize something. I had no control over so much of it, but organization gives me a sense of control and that there are things I can do to make my life easier and make other people's lives easier. Discipline was a strength that carried me through this "journey" we call breast cancer. I organized my diagnosis information, doctor's appointment notes, treatment and medication details into multiple notebooks. When I started feeling a little bit better, I realized how close I was to death. I didn't want to die and have my daughters flounder around looking for everything they needed like I had to do when my mother passed. I'm a collector and have a lot of stuff

that's really important to me. Now, I realize it probably doesn't mean a hoot to my kids, but I don't want to get rid of it while I'm alive. When I'm gone, I want them to know the history of these things and why it was important to me before they get rid of it. I put together this binder with my insurance policies, my wills, the endowments we've set up with different organizations, and pictures and notes of my collections that have meaning to me. I have pictures of my grandmother's crystal, family jewelry, and special gifts. I cataloged each item and wrote a note of the history, like "This diamond was important to me because it was the first diamond your father gave to me." The girls are thrilled that I did that because it will make their life a lot easier.[40]

Make the space your own

Be aware of your surroundings and how they are impacting your mood and energy levels. I associate this strength with the practice of minimalism as people with this strength often keep clean neat spaces, including their homes, desks, and cars. Cancer centers are fairly simple, sterile, and bland. If you need something to make the space feel more comfortable for you, consider bringing a blanket, small plant, framed picture, or personal keepsake. Use your talent of creating order to help you design your desired atmosphere or vibe in the spaces where you'll be spending your time.

Are your planning tools fit for purpose?

You embrace systems, tools, and perhaps technology to create your routines and schedules. Are there any tools that would help your cancer planning? This is a major life disruption for you and will need to be accounted for as you plan your time in the future months and potentially years. What has helped you feel in control of your time in the past?

---

40 McCausland, T., *Follow Your Strengths*, (2021). "Discipline: Sharon Juon." Available at: https://www.followyourstrengths.com/blog/achiever-jen-slabas-guidi-9msly-tw2p2-4llj7-hd7n7.

Do you gravitate toward planners, software, or apps? Consider asking your care team, other cancer survivors, or conducting online research to find realistic timelines and tools that might be helpful for you to incorporate into your planning process.

Avoid avoidable surprises
Ask your care providers how long appointments, treatments, and side effects typically last. For example, do you need to only block out your morning or will certain treatments or appointments take a longer chunk of time? The more *knowns* that can be created during this unknown process for you, the better you will be able to plan. You don't like surprises. You don't like not knowing what to expect or how your schedule will be impacted.

Plan your document and data management strategy
Create a strategy for how you will keep track of the medical information you'll be consuming in the weeks and months ahead. Doing so will be calming to you because you'll feel more in control. Examples include appointment details, insurance information, billing statements, and cancer-related handouts or pamphlets.

If you prefer paper documents and holding information in your hands, invest in a physical file folder organizer, binder, or file cabinet. If you gravitate toward electronic storage of information, use a reliable source such as your phone, computer, or tablet. Your medical notes and results, such as labs and imaging, will be stored electronically on a patient portal at your medical center. Bookmark the web page so you can find it easily.

Initially, I carried a purple file folder with me to my appointments and filled it with handouts and printouts. Shortly into my chemotherapy, I realized I didn't need to bring this with me anymore. Instead, I transitioned to brainstorming and typing questions for my oncologist or surgeon into the Notes app on my phone. I found this to be efficient and easily accessible for me and preferable to paper and pen.

Be prepared for schedule alterations

You are timely and typically finish things before their due date. Cancer treatment is often a story of missed deadlines and shifting timelines. Be meticulously organized as you always are and take comfort in your Discipline strength, not because the outcome is perfect but because you are taking care of yourself.

Set the expectation that the best-laid plans may still need to shift, so you consider that part of the plan. Be prepared to work with your frustration when timelines flex since so many variables are at play, such as physician and operating room schedules, your blood count, and side effects that may lead to delays. Other examples are procedure availability such as MRIs, X-rays, genetic testing, and CT scans. The coordination and scheduling of people, procedures, and resources is complex with many moving pieces and delays and snafus are inevitable. Consider how you've successfully handled delays in other situations, and work to replicate that approach here.

Be proactive

Your precision and follow-through may not be noticed or honored in the medical system automatically, so work to position these qualities to your advantage. For example, you may have to get labs drawn and complete multiple online documents prior to scheduling your next appointment. Complete your pre-work early and be proactive by calling instead of waiting to be contacted. This initiative on your part delivers no guarantees of reduced waiting times for you, but it does honor your desire to finish things early and be prepared if an opportunity exists. You may love the saying "Success occurs when preparation meets opportunity." When opportunities emerge that can positively impact your health outcomes, you will be prepared. Additionally, a cancer center or care provider that meets your needs for efficiency and timeliness is perfectly acceptable as part of your evaluation criteria.

Cancer Cautions

Be open to new ideas
It is very rare for someone to have both Discipline and Ideation as top strengths. If you are in that majority where your Discipline strength is higher than Ideation, consider what creative options you could be missing or dismissing. Given your preference for establishing a plan and meticulously following it, remind yourself to be open to new ideas, suggestions, and resources. They may not have been part of your original treatment plan, but that doesn't mean they aren't valid and worthy of consideration. You may meet new cancer survivors or care team members who share interesting research, statistics, or advice based on their experience. Ignoring new or novel information keeps your original plan in place; however, it doesn't mean that you're still following the best plan. Imagine that your cancer plan is written in pencil rather than permanent marker.

If you feel impatient, take the long view
You operate best when you know what the schedule is and can anticipate deadlines. Especially in the early days and weeks of diagnosis and establishing your treatment plan, timelines and expectations may not come as quickly as you'd like—and that uncertainty can be stressful for you. The waiting game can be brutal, even for people without this strength of Discipline. Assure yourself that the initial waiting process helps to ensure a more effective and smooth care plan in the long run.

Anticipate some disorganization
You are likely more organized than most people you encounter. Keep this in mind as you move through the cancer world. Remind yourself to expect delays, hiccups, and mistakes along the way. Instead of letting the unpredictable approach of others frustrate you, try to focus on the outcomes and big picture. That is ultimately what matters much more than how somebody checks you in for chemo or if you get out of the parking garage in the most efficient manner. If you anticipate delays and lack of

organization from some of the people and processes you encounter, then your experience will feel less disappointing and more like things went as you had planned.

Empathy

People exceptionally talented in the Empathy theme have an instinctive ability to understand people. They feel others' emotions as if they were their own.

I'd always thought my Empathy strength was focused externally and on the feelings of others. When I was diagnosed, I quickly realized I needed to turn that strength inward, stay in tune with my feelings, and give myself some grace.

—Jen, melanoma survivor

You can sense the emotions of those around you. Intuitively, you feel what they are feeling as though their feelings are your own. You do not necessarily agree with each person's perspective, feel pity for their predicament, or condone their choices, but you do understand. This instinctive ability to understand is powerful. You hear the unasked questions. You anticipate the needs. When people struggle to express their feelings—to themselves and to others—you seem to find the right words and the right tone. You give voice to their emotions. For all these reasons, people are drawn to you.

Characteristics of Those with Empathy Talents

Listening	Emotional	Expressive
Sensitive	Aware	Intuitive
Confidential	Helpful	Sensate

Cancer Connection

Your intuitive nature and ability to sense what others are feeling will be a valuable strength as you navigate cancer and all the related emotions. Pay close attention to what people and places energize you and your emotional battery. Intentionally build those beneficial experiences into your days. Likewise, some places and people will drain you and exhaust your emotions. Make sure you have some strategies that help you recover from challenging places and create boundaries to protect yourself from people who negatively impact your health and well-being.

As we discuss throughout this book, there's no shortage of information available for most cancers. In fact, some may argue there's too much information available since some of it is inaccurate and even dangerous. That said, you're able to draw on an additional source of information that many cannot access as effortlessly. You easily see, hear, and notice emotions from others by how they appear, what they say, and even what they don't say. This intuitiveness gives you a great advantage as you approach cancer from a place of openness and awareness.

As you gather information from other cancer survivors, you will easily be able to sense and feel how they experience life as a survivor. Keep in mind that you do not have to feel the same way as others. Some survivors are grateful for the clarity cancer provided, others angry it wasn't caught sooner, and others calm and rational about it being just one chapter of their life. It's valuable to hear different perspectives, but you don't have to feel any of those exact sentiments. It reinforces what you already know—people's emotions are real, valid, temporary, and unique.

Cancer Considerations

Ensure you have good support

You may feel emotions strongly and you may experience a variety of feelings after being diagnosed with cancer. These can range from:
- Shock to denial to guilt
- Fear to anger to sadness
- Tiredness to annoyance to frustration
- Gratitude to appreciation to thankfulness
- Joy to relief to celebration

That is a lot to navigate, especially since you may experience most of these varying emotions within a matter of days. Make sure you have at least one person who you can count on to process through your emotions. Request a referral to a counselor or psychologist from your medical team or join a reputable local or virtual support group so someone can support you. It's important to let in help during this time so you can focus some of your empathy on yourself and your healing.

Protect your emotions

Be prepared when you enter a cancer center. Some of what you will see in the waiting rooms and hallways may be difficult, including patients who are younger than you or patients clearly nearing the end of their lives. You may see patients with an eager support system that looks simultaneously encouraging and terrified. You will see people who are alone. I remember sitting in the infusion center waiting area with a few of my best friends when a prison guard wheeled an inmate into the room, wearing handcuffs and leg chains. This new patient caught the attention of most of us but likely had more impact on the empathetic patients in the room. In that scenario, you might wonder about that person's transfer to the hospital, their experience of standing out, and what facing cancer from prison is like. When you are getting treatment, remind yourself to separate your emotions from those swirling around you and remain focused on your health.

Balance facts with emotions
Your decision-making process may be more feelings-based and emotion-driven than cancer survivors with other strengths. While checking in with your feelings is a smart approach and one you will always do, make sure you are also considering facts, data, and logic to make health care choices. Tell your care team and supporters "Help me consider the objective portion of this decision, as I've already considered the emotional side."

Be a wet dog
If your emotions about your cancer become difficult to handle, make sure you have a couple of outlets for releasing these feelings. Reach out to a trusted friend or family member who is a great listener. Engage in your favorite form of exercise and movement. Get outside in nature and focus on your breathing. In a conversation with a therapist years ago, she asked me if I thought I was an empath. She described how empaths may absorb the feelings around them and she recommended "shaking them off like a dog shakes off water." Try being a wet dog once a day to free yourself and make space for your healing.

You may be your own best resource
When sharing your cancer diagnosis news with friends, family and colleagues, you will instantly be able to sense how they are feeling about your news. While they will undoubtedly want to lend you support, keep in mind that you may have a better skillset in this arena than they do, and you may be your own best resource.

Jen, a cancer survivor from Washington, D.C., shared, "I'd always thought my Empathy strength was focused externally and on the feelings of others. When I was diagnosed, I quickly realized I needed to turn that strength inward, stay in tune with my feelings, and give myself some grace as I navigated this rare melanoma diagnosis."

Be open to letting your supporters help you
Be open to engaging your support system and asking for help. Two survivors shared how they let their friends get involved. Michelle commented,

"I know how weird it feels when you just don't know what to do for somebody. So, I let my friends have a party in my honor. I knew it would be helpful for them." Another survivor, Deb, commented, "I'm struggling with this diagnosis, and I know they are too. It made me feel better to ask others for help because it gave them a sense of contributing."

Create a space you can control
Consider creating a space that reflects how you'd like to feel as you deal with cancer. If you desire more peace and calm in your life, add a candle near your bathtub or dedicate a shelf in your closet for rejuvenation and relaxation products. If you'd like to focus on time for quiet and reflection, make a cozy corner for reading or meditating. Carve out a space for stretching or lifting light weights. Since you won't always be able to control the environments in the hospital or clinics, work to control what you can in the spaces you occupy most often at work and at home.

Cancer Cautions

You are not responsible for how people feel
Just because you can sense the emotions of others doesn't mean you need to take any ownership of their feelings. A cancer diagnosis creates an intense, stressful experience for those closely involved. You do not have to carry the emotions of other adults or feel obligated to fix or troubleshoot their difficult feelings. Your health and emotions need to be center stage and your primary focus.

Be alert to the need for boundaries
You may sense that your support team is shocked and saddened by your diagnosis, which is natural. Although you are typically the one providing a listening ear and affirming feelings, don't expect yourself to comfort others as they experience their emotions about your news. In fact, there may be some people whose actions or words physically drain you. Be

prepared to set boundaries to limit those interactions. You need to, for your own well-being.

Get the facts from your care team
You'll be spending a lot of time with medical professionals. You are a natural at reading between the lines, but don't try to do that with your care team. Be careful not to jump to conclusions on what they are thinking or feeling about your treatment. Instead, ask clarifying questions and make them state clearly what they think or suggest.

Focus

People exceptionally talented in the Focus theme can take a direction, follow through and make the corrections necessary to stay on track. They prioritize, then act.

> Letting go of what I can't control was one of the biggest lessons of cancer. It taught me not to take on the problems of the world.
>
> —Melissa, breast cancer survivor

"Where am I headed?" You ask yourself this every day. Without a clear destination, your life and your work can quickly become frustrating. So you set goals that serve as your compass, helping you determine priorities and make corrections to stay on course. Your Focus compels you to filter— to instinctively evaluate if a particular action will help you move toward your goal. If it doesn't, you ignore it. You are efficient. You can become impatient with delays, obstacles, and tangents. In your mind, if something is not helping you move toward your destination, then it is not important. And if it is not important, then it is not worth your time. You keep everyone on point.

Characteristics of Those with Focus Talents

Goal-oriented	Driven	Single-minded
Selective	Persevering	Progress-aware
Efficient	Distraction-averse	

Cancer Connection

A cancer diagnosis often brings life into sharp focus for people. You already see life, goals, and priorities with distinct clarity. Receiving a cancer diagnosis will feel like a deviation from the path you were on before this life disruption, but your Focus strength will help you tremendously. In the early days or weeks of your diagnosis, however, you will have to make an intentional effort to recalibrate. What you were focusing on and driving toward before may not need to go away entirely, but some priorities and deadlines may need to shift due to the amount of time you are spending in medical appointments, researching your options, and making decisions.

Your Focus strength will help you when you meet with your medical team. Their time is often limited during these appointments, and you will not waste it with small talk or getting off topic. They will appreciate this, and you will be energized by the efficient cadence of these medical conversations.

Your perseverance and commitment to your goals will guide you through cancer. You may experience side effects of treatment, unexpected setbacks, or challenges with delays or disruptions in your care. These detours can derail some cancer survivors and lead them to spiral into negative thoughts. With your Focus strength, you know that sometimes plans go off track and you also know that you have the determination to get them back on track. Your care team members and supporters will be impressed by your perseverance, grit, and determination to focus in on your one goal—improving your health.

Cancer Considerations

Keep sight of the big picture
You will do a great job of keeping the big picture of your cancer treatment plan at the forefront. For example, you may not get too rattled when your sleep schedule is briefly disrupted from the steroid they pair with your chemotherapy drug. As you're wide awake at 2 a.m., you spend more time thinking this will help remove or reduce the impact of cancer on your body than you do worrying about those few extra hours of sleep.

Review your commitments
Your commitments are important to you. Evaluate what you've committed to and what's currently on your plate. Look closely at your work projects, community involvement, and family obligations to determine what may need to be modified given the increased load on your calendar with medical appointments. Consider reducing or removing some obligations as you focus time and energy on your health.

Audit your time
Time and place will be important for you to maintain your Focus strength. What time of day do you feel your sharpest? What is the best environment for you to get things accomplished with less effort? Try to replicate what worked best for you before your cancer diagnosis and be willing to shift if your body is telling you something needs to change. For example, you may have been the most alert and productive in the early afternoon prior to your cancer diagnosis. But after chemotherapy treatments, you may realize that now the afternoon brings fatigue and foggy thinking, so try shifting your key hours for making progress on work or other projects to the morning instead of early afternoon. This may be a process of trial and error, but well worth it when you find that ideal sweet spot again.

Define some new goals
You are driven and goal-oriented. What new goals can you create related to your cancer diagnosis, treatment plan, or overall health and well-being?

If exercise is an important component for reducing the risk of recurrence for your kind of cancer, you may create a goal for the number of minutes you walk weekly or the number of steps you take daily. While some cancer survivors may say they are going to do this, you will not only say it, but you will plan it, do it, and track it.

Dr. Melissa Reade shared a couple of great tools that helped during her breast cancer experience. She leveraged her professional experience, including her role as executive director of a nonprofit called Leader Valley, her FranklinCovey certification, and her years as an educator and principal in developing her cancer strategy. She used FranklinCovey's 30/10 approach[41] for her weekly planning and would spend 30 minutes on Sunday making her plans for the week. Each day of the week, she would spend 10 minutes and revisit her plan asking herself, "What do I need to do today to help move these things forward?" As Melissa evaluated different activities, she asked herself, "Will this help me beat cancer?" She was careful to only allow those items in her plan, and the rest would not get her focus. This led her to reducing outside commitments, such as evening events, to conserve her energy levels. She also created a NOT-To-Do List where she carefully spelled out activities or behaviors that drained her energy or weakened her spirit. Examples on her NOT-To-Do List are "Say yes to every person selling something" and "Be indecisive and let others make choices for me."

Additionally, Melissa leveraged the Circle of Influence® concept[42] from Stephen Covey's book *The 7 Habits of Highly Effective People*[43] and was careful not to put her energy toward things she couldn't control. Another cancer survivor agreed, sharing that "Letting go of what I can't control was one of the biggest lessons of cancer. It taught me not to take

---

41 FranklinCovey (undated). The 5 Choices to Extraordinary Productivity®, "Choice 3: Schedule the Big Rocks, Don't Sort Gravel®." Available at: https://www.franklincovey.com/courses/the-5-choices/choice-3.

42 FranklinCovey (undated). "Habit 1: Be Proactive." *The 7 Habits of Highly Effective People*®. Available at: https://www.franklincovey.com/the-7-habits/habit-1.

43 Covey, S. (1989). *The 7 Habits of Highly Effective People*. 30th anniversary ed. 2020. Simon & Schuster.

on the problems of the world." The 30/10 planning approach, NOT-To-Do List, and Circle of Influence® are all tools Melissa continues to leverage, years after her cancer diagnosis.

Cancer Cautions

Avoid seeing cancer as your only focus
Cancer doesn't have to be your only focus. Depending on the kind of cancer and the severity of your prognosis, it may feel more like a distraction to you than a new major element of your life.

Be flexible
Some of your previous goals may need to shift. Do not think of this as failing to meet your goals. Think of it as adjusting as circumstances change. Any big goals you've met in your life prior to this most likely involved a few challenges, setbacks, and adjustments. In those situations, you probably didn't enjoy adjusting either, but you did it, and still hit your goal. Take that approach with you as you navigate your new cancer and health-related goals.

Futuristic

People exceptionally talented in the Futuristic theme vividly imagine the future. They inspire and energize others with their vision of what could be.

You live for the future. Often, you are already there. You are a dreamer who loves to peer over the horizon. As if it were projected on the wall, you see in detail what the future might hold, and it keeps pulling you forward into tomorrow. While exactly what you see depends on your other strengths and interests—a better product, a better team, a better life, or a better world—it will always inspire you. When the present is too frustrating, your visions of the future energize you. They can energize others too. When you describe the possibilities and potential you see to other people, be as vivid as possible. Your forward-looking ideas can inspire them. People are drawn to the hope you bring.

I just know your mind and imagination is powerful. I future-paced. I told myself, "I am strong, healthy, and whole. I'm living long, long, long on this earth.

—*Amy, breast cancer survivor*

Characteristics of Those with Futuristic Talents

Creative	Anticipating	Communicating
Inspiring	Imaginative	Perceptive
Vivid	Expressive	Future-oriented

Cancer Connection

Your natural state and where you feel best is when you're imagining and anticipating the future. Whereas those with Futuristic as a lesser strength may be dwelling on the potential cause of their cancer or devastated by each phase of the treatment process, you are naturally inclined to be looking ahead and dreaming about what could be. This is absolutely a unique advantage that will give you a mental edge as you move through your cancer experience. Of course, your vision for your future may shift based on your diagnosis, so be prepared to adjust the initial plan. Deb, a 10-year two-time breast cancer survivor shared, "I had a strong vision there was a future me. It was very rare for me to get really discouraged; not to say it didn't happen. But I could see myself down the road and that helped tremendously."

Your Futuristic talents give you energy when imagining the future and what could be. When your supporters are around you, they probably feel more positive, optimistic, and hopeful for the future. Work to anticipate where you may need assistance during your treatment and recovery. People are turning to you to see how they can help make any of your visions a reality. Delegate some tasks to people who can help turn your dreams into actions, from larger initiatives at work to smaller projects at your house that will help you feel inspired.

A nurse in the cancer clinic gave me the advice to think about the treatment path like climbing a mountain. When you're at the bottom, you can barely see the top and the climb looks nearly impossible, like reaching the estimated "end" of your cancer treatment. She encouraged me to realize there would be many mini milestones along the way. This was helpful for me to hear as I was overwhelmed by the amount of time required for my treatment plan.

Futuristic is low on my CliftonStrengths talent profile. I see time from two different standpoints: now and not now. This is not a gift. When I initially received my cancer diagnosis, the priority was to understand my immediate treatment plan and next steps. We were informed that my medical path would begin with chemotherapy, followed by a month break, and conclude with surgery and potentially radiation. The length of my treatment was six to eight months, followed by five years of daily medication.

This length of treatment felt like an eternity based on how I process time. I don't know what I'm doing next Friday, let alone eight months from now. Given my work around strengths, it struck me early on that the Futuristic strength would be very helpful on the front end of a cancer diagnosis to process the time necessary to endure treatment and survivorship. Your creative imagination may be one of your greatest assets from the day of your diagnosis, forward. Your effortless ability to dream and envision a better future will serve as a tremendous complementary therapy during your cancer experience.

Cancer Considerations

Help your team help you see further
If you are driven to understand your diagnosis and medical journey deeply, ask your healthcare team great questions about your next steps and potential implications of current research on your disease, treatment, and recovery process. You have an ability to challenge current state thinking which means you can push your medical team to think further down the road than most patients. Ask questions about clinical trials, exciting research underway, cutting-edge technology, and other medical advancements related to your diagnosis. Use this gift as you and your medical team explore treatment options and recovery plans.

Think big, imagine, and stay curious

You are energized by anticipating the future and may be known for your impressive imagination. Think of examples of how you used this strength in the years leading up to your diagnosis, like the creative project you started at your local food bank, how you anticipated the upcoming needs of your teenager, or the proactive pivot you took in your small business. Remind yourself of those moments, and continue using this strength to think big, imagine, and stay curious as you progress through treatment and survivorship. Create a visual to show what's left of your current phase or the entire treatment process. This visual will help you look forward to what's ahead.

Imagine the ideal future

You are often able to paint the picture or visualize where things are headed without getting too stuck in where they are today. Challenge yourself to look beyond the pain or limitations when you are having a rough day. Tap into your dreams and visions for the future, whether that is weeks, months, or years from now. You might journal about things you're looking forward to when your health improves, such as taking a trip, learning a new language, or increasing your daily number of steps or intensity of your hikes. Simply the act of imagining the future will provide you with a much-needed energy boost. You are comfortable living in the future so let that view bring you peace.

Amy is a four-year breast cancer survivor, a mother of two, a powerhouse realtor, and a pillar of her community. When she received the shocking news of her breast cancer diagnosis, she instinctively knew she needed to look at herself in her ideal state. Amy shared, "I just know your mind and imagination is so powerful. I was very careful with what would come out of my mouth. Even though I may have been experiencing fear, I never took ownership. So, I declared every day, 'I am strong, healthy, and whole. I'm living long, long, long on this earth.'" Amy's Futuristic strength means she is strong in visualizing. Early in her diagnosis, Amy shared that she future-paced. She looked at pictures from before her diagnosis where she looked healthy and created a photo of herself with her kids on a boat—way in the future when she looked really old. It was a reminder to her that "I'm living long and strong in my life. I'm going to be old and taking my kids on fantastic vacations." She placed visual reminders of hope, and photos of her strong and healthy, in places where she would see them daily like her bookbag, office, and car console. These were powerful images that helped Amy shift her emotions and anchor herself in the future, rather than getting sucked into the cold and fearful feelings tied to the cancer clinic and radiation rooms.

Waiting time is also dreaming time

One thing that is common across all types of cancer is the waiting game. Many cancer survivors spend hundreds and potentially thousands of hours in waiting rooms, infusion chairs, radiation oncology clinics, and surgery centers. You need to plan for this downtime to avoid frustration and boredom. Because of your Futuristic strength, you could use this idle time as your planning, scheming, and dreaming time. You have loved thinking about the future since you were young. In assigning a purpose to this inevitable downtime, it can energize you and create a feeling of forward momentum. You can also use this time to refine your dreams, aiming for more color, clarity, and actions that will make your visions a reality. Capture your visions. Write them down. Draw them. Make a video. Talk about them with your family, friends, and colleagues.

Connect with other futurists

Your present situation may be tiring, painful, and extremely challenging. Focusing on the current state may drain or depress you. Reach out and engage with other futurists and dreamers to improve your mood and energy. Are there people you know personally who inspire you with their vision? Are there thought leaders, books, movies, and podcasts that fuel your forward-seeking tendencies? You're looking for ways to give yourself a mental edge and lean into this strength. These activities may not take your pain away, but they should give you an energy boost as you work through your challenging reality.

Zero in on hope

Think beyond your current medical challenges to your future health and well-being. Can you be hopeful for things related to the people in your life or for your future plans and desires? Are you hopeful for your current circles, whether that's your family, employer, faith and spiritual community, or your broader community as a whole? What progress and hope do you see for those groups, and are there any small actions you can take now to work toward those visions?

Cancer Cautions

Notice the good things about today

While you may always have been more likely to look toward the future than live in the present moment, your cancer diagnosis may have intensified that desire. Are there great moments and experiences you're missing today? Can you glean some positive momentum out of things happening in the here-and-now? Even though you are dealing with cancer, which clouds the present, your life still has moments of beauty and joy. Pay attention and use that positive energy to grow your gratitude and propel you forward.

Don't overlook the current state

Given your forward-looking bent, you may have already mentally moved on to the next step in your healing. For example, you may have recently been diagnosed but you're already thinking about finishing your treatment. Or you may be undergoing chemotherapy yet focused on your next treatment phase of radiation. Doing this could mean missing recommendations and strategies for your current phase of treatment that would improve your future outcomes. Be intentional about remaining present for certain conversations and decisions. Work to stay engaged so you can be fully informed. Leverage your support system as you prepare for appointments to help you brainstorm questions and capture actions that need your immediate attention.

Anticipate milestones

Some cancer survivors struggle emotionally as they face certain milestones. You tend to naturally think ahead, so do your best to anticipate these milestones. Examples include your diagnosis date, surgery date, certain annual events such as birthdays, holidays, or seasons that trigger cancer memories. If you anticipate that a milestone is going to bother you, make a plan in advance. Some people like to create distractions for themselves by staying busy that day or scheduling a fun activity with friends or family to serve as a positive intervention. You may choose to ignore the date completely or honor it by acknowledging it as a major achievement in your life.

Share your fears

Another common challenge cancer survivors face involves worrying about future checkups, which may include scans, lab work, and exams. Many refer to this feeling as "scanxiety." According to a research article published by the National Institute of Health, "Scanxiety represents a complex array of negative and stressful emotions linked with cancer scans and the uncertainties and fears that may accompany them."[44] If you are struggling with fear and anxiety related to what's ahead, consider sharing this with your medical provider, talking it through with friends or family, joining a support group, or engaging with a counselor. Additionally, bring calm into your life by simply slowing down or exploring physical interventions such as meditation, stretching, yoga, and deep breathing exercises. Schedule other activities that feel relaxing to you, such as reading, hiking, or coffee with a friend, during the time of your peak anxiety.

Monitor your mental health

From the day you heard the words "You have cancer," your life outlook may have shifted. Some survivors take a one-day-at-a time approach to

---

44 Derry-Vick, H. M. and others, National Institute of Health, National Library of Medicine, "Scanxiety Among Adults with Cancer: A Scoping Review to Guide Research and Interventions." Available at: https://www.ncbi.nlm.nih.gov/pmc/articles/PMC10000102.

their cancer experience, but you are likely looking at the bigger picture with a longer, telephoto lens. As you process statistics, percentages, and prognosis details from your care team, some level of fear and anxiety is normal. Do not let this invoke paralyzing fear in you. Stay in tune with your mental health and your fear of recurrence or even death, depending on your disease stage and prognosis. Consider engaging help from medical professionals with counseling and therapy if thoughts of the future overwhelm, depress, or no longer energize you as they did historically.

Harmony

People exceptionally talented in the Harmony theme look for consensus. They have no use for unnecessary friction and guide others toward practical solutions.

You look for areas of agreement. In your view, there is little to gain from conflict and friction, so you try to keep them to a minimum. Always looking for common ground, you steer people with different views away from confrontation and toward consensus. When others strongly express their fervently held beliefs, claims, and opinions, you hold your peace. When others make a decision, you instinctively modify your objectives to merge with theirs, as long as their values do not clash with yours. When others are locked in disagreement, you can help unlock them. You can't quite believe how much time people waste trying to impose their views on others. You have no use for unnecessary arguments. Instead, you know that focusing on practical matters that everyone can agree on is more productive.

Our hardest challenge was sharing the news with our two young boys, just 9 and 4 at that time. My husband and I both have Harmony, and I believe we delivered the news in a calm, stable, and loving way.

Characteristics of Those with Harmony Talents

Practical	Conflict-reducing	Agreeable
Concrete	Collaborative	Task-oriented

Cancer Connection

People with Harmony as a strength tend to be calm, logical, and practical. You are likely very skilled at seeking out opinions of experts and relying on their insights and feedback before making decisions. This skillset will be beneficial for you in understanding the current state of your health and evaluating your care options. When you work in small groups, teams, or committees, your vibe is one of collaboration, curiosity, and cohesion. Bring this presence with you as you become the captain of your care team's circle and conversations.

You tend to value efficiency and forward movement through projects, even when conflict arises, or especially when conflict arises. You're not one to dwell on differences or simmer in drama, so you will take this practical approach to cancer too. What drama can cancer deliver? Fair question. Your initial consultation with an oncologist may be rescheduled, your surgeon may quit and leave the institution, or your child may be upset because you are too tired for the weekend bike ride you promised. While some cancer patients may opt to call and yell at the receptionist about the reschedule or the surgeon quitting, you instinctively know these are situations beyond your or the receptionist's control and you won't waste your energy. A crying child may send another survivor into a tailspin of sadness, but you know that it's just one day and you offer to read their favorite bedtime story instead. Your ability to artfully meet people in the middle through calm negotiations will help you along the way.

Your cancer experience may also include difficult conversations, differing medical opinions, and challenging decisions. Be sure to leverage your Harmony strength as you work through these moments with your care team, family, and supporters. For example, you may make a medical decision that a colleague questions or hear different advice from two survivors about which hospital to select. Our hardest challenge was sharing the news with our two young boys, just 9 and 4 at that time. We opted to wait until we understood what my treatment path would entail, and this allowed us to get our oldest son closer to the end of the school year. Prior to telling them, we had a meeting with their amazing school principal and counselor. Mrs. Hart and Mrs. Squires were such blessings to us during that stressful time and helped guide us on the best way and timing for sharing this news. We will never forget their empathetic support. My husband and I both have Harmony within our top three strengths, and I believe we delivered the news to the boys in a calm, stable, and loving way. There were a few tears, but they felt confident that we were in incredible hands with the care team at UIHC. Within 15 minutes of sharing our news, Jay was off to his buddy Cason's house, and I got a text from his mom. She said, "He told us within the first five minutes. He said she is going to have treatments and will use wigs and hats. I'm not sure how you presented it to him," she went on, "but it must have been perfect. What a challenge for parents to say the right words, but clearly you did." This feedback reassured us that Jay received this difficult news in the calm way we intended.

Remind yourself to reduce areas of potential friction where you can and continue to move through these moments in your usual grounded way. Your Harmony strength is active, and you won't let it become complacent or checked out. Ask great questions, listen closely, distill the information you receive to its essence, and make the best decision for you. Your approach to these challenges will amaze your supporters and likely help bring them closer to your levelheaded approach, which is a win for all.

Cancer Considerations

Your decisions will be balanced
You are skilled in truly listening to different perspectives. Remind yourself of this strength as you consider different care centers, physicians,

and treatment options. You will probably hear many different survivor stories. You will know to take their stories for what they are—just one example of just one person. This neutral approach comes easily to you and will allow you to create effective pro/con lists on paper that will serve your decision-making process well.

Your approach is calm and practical

You are known for being calm, steady, and anchored. While your cancer diagnosis may shake you and disrupt your world, your practical mindset will help you remain focused on reality and the immediate tasks at hand. You may tell yourself and others things like "I feel really good about the preliminary surgery results but won't celebrate until we receive the official pathology results next week," or "We aren't going to worry about worst-case scenarios until those are in play."

You set the tone for reaction

Sharing the news of your cancer diagnosis can be difficult, and the level of difficulty can range depending on many factors including your prognosis, age at diagnosis, family history of the disease, and impact on other people such as young children or work associates. You will no doubt do a great job of handling the daunting task of telling others but may still sense that people are more emotional and distraught than you. While it is not your job to calm your family, friends, or colleagues, keep in mind that your steady approach will ripple out to your supporters. Be conscious of the calming energy you bring to a group and describe your feelings out loud if you'd like a shared understanding of your current cancer emotions. Your smooth delivery of the news will set the tone for your supporters.

Create a serene space for yourself

You enjoy equilibrium, calmness, and agreement. Picture an arrangement of Zen stacked rocks; a beautiful body of smooth water; or your hands folded in the Hindu greeting *namaste*, a common yoga phrase. How can you create a space that honors your calm preference? Can you add an element of serenity to your bedroom, office, or another place you spend your time? I created this vibe on our screened-in porch with a small fountain I bought when I began chemotherapy. I loved spending my summer days either working a few hours on the porch, relaxing and reading, or visiting with friends when they stopped by to check in on me. Even though I was bald and tired, the fresh air all around me and the soothing sounds of the fountain in the background supported my healing process as a reminder to stay calm and breathe.

Visualize your care providers as your team
You are probably known for being a team player or "the glue" that holds a group together. Rather than thinking of your providers as separate players, consciously think of them as your official care team. Visualize your oncologist, radiologist, surgeon, physical therapist, psychologist, pharmacist, and general practitioner wearing the same color uniforms with your name on the back. Many of them communicate frequently and already know they are teammates in your care, but some may simply receive updates through your electronic records. The visualization and verbalization to them being on the same team will boost your confidence in your treatment.

Cancer Cautions

Assess whether you have considered all options
With your desire to make decisions based on what is known and not "rock the boat," as the CliftonStrengths assessment states, you may frustrate people who prefer to question and investigate current medical practices. Before moving forward with healthcare decisions, check in with yourself to see if there are other possibilities worth considering. Is there a care center worth contacting to arrange for a second opinion beyond the nearby center where it would be easiest to receive treatment? Is there a new product or procedure worth talking to an expert about before you rule it out? Check in before you finalize care decisions to be sure you've remained open to new ideas or options.

It's hard to make a decision in the absence of consensus

During your diagnosis and treatment phases, you may hear conflicting opinions. For example, one oncologist may recommend a different path forward than another at a different center. One surgeon may recommend an aggressive procedure, whereas another plays it more conservatively. I encountered a very difficult decision immediately following the best news ever. After completing five months of neoadjuvant chemotherapy and double mastectomy surgery, I achieved a pathologic complete response (pCR).[45] This essentially meant that all tissue removed during surgery showed no signs of cancer and that chemotherapy worked. Although this may sound common, the excitement in the voices of my oncologist and breast surgeon said otherwise when they each phoned me with the news. The odds of receiving a pCR for women with the same kind of tumors I had was only 10%, which helped explain my doctors' joy.

Just after receiving the best news ever, I then faced an extremely difficult decision. My initial treatment plan included radiation; however, the incredible pCR outcome blurred the lines and radiation could be erased from my original plan. Essentially, I could walk out of the follow-up appointment with my oncologist and begin my five years on tamoxifen, a daily pill that blocks estrogen. At that time, there was no evidence showing that adding radiation after pCR would increase my survival rate or decrease recurrence. There was a clinical trial underway, but the data wouldn't be available for at least seven years. I requested a radiology consult to learn more and, not surprisingly, that physician strongly recommended I should still do radiation. Ugh.

We were faced with two options, and essentially no wrong decision based on the available information. Choosing a side when there is no consensus of opinion is a stressful process for somebody with the Harmony strength. It paralyzed me for three days. I was filled with uncertainty, doubt, and second-guessing. I reached out to Dr. Phadke and Dr.

---

45 Pathologic complete response (pCR) definition, NCI Dictionary of Cancer Terms: https://www.cancer.gov/publications/dictionaries/cancer-terms/def/pathologic-complete-response.

Sugg, my oncologist and surgeon, and they took my unique pCR case to their weekly Tumor Board, a multidisciplinary team that meets weekly to review new and complex scenarios.[46] I ultimately decided to not do radiation due to the lack of data saying it would help somebody with pCR. My decision had support from the Tumor Board. To this day, I do not regret this decision. And to this day, stirring in those conflicting opinions and weighing them against the unknown for three days was one of the toughest stretches of my cancer experience.

---

46 Tumor Boards, Holden Comprehensive Cancer Care: https://cancer.uiowa.edu/tumor-boards.

Ideation

People exceptionally talented in the Ideation theme are fascinated by ideas. They see connections that others don't and can view the world from different perspectives.

> I used my Ideation strength to come up with ideas on how to best manage each day. This ensured I continued to live a meaningful, joyful existence, so much so that many friends were surprised when I shared I was going through a cancer journey.
>
> —Catherine, breast cancer survivor

You are fascinated by ideas. When you discover an elegantly simple explanation for a complex situation, you are delighted. With a mind that is always looking for connections, you are intrigued when seemingly unrelated events or circumstances are somehow linked to each other. You take the world we know and turn it around so we can see it from a new perspective. You love ideas because they explain, because they clarify, because they connect, and because they challenge you to reimagine the familiar. For all these reasons, you get a jolt of energy whenever a new idea occurs to you.

Characteristics of Those with Ideation Talents

Spontaneous   Innovative   Artistic
Creative   Collaborative   Insightful

Cancer Connection

People with Ideation as a strength love spontaneity and originality. You are probably creative, innovative, and energized by exploring ideas. Is there a way you can take this style of yours along with you as you move through your cancer experience? Can you be a creative cancer survivor and approach your experience uniquely?

As you sit with your cancer diagnosis and consider your options, spend some time thinking about your Ideation strength. Reflect on your life and how you've used this strength in the past to come up with new and creative ideas. Does this happen to you when you brainstorm and ideate with others or when you spend time alone? Do ideas come to you when you're talking out loud, journaling and writing, or sitting in solitude? Cancer might not seem like an area for creativity, but your Ideation successes and wins over the years may reveal some patterns that you can use through this challenging experience. Dig into those themes and work to replicate them with your health and well-being decisions moving forward.

Your mind is typically looking for connections between ideas, people, and events. Most cancer diagnoses involve multiple appointments, steps, and phases of treatment. Given the way you are innately looking for connections, it will be helpful for you to understand how all phases of your treatment plan come together. If the initial plan shifts or changes, ask your care team to help you regroup and reorient to the new plan. A cancer diagnosis typically creates a variety of new thoughts, ideas, and questions regardless of a person's top strengths. Given your strength of Ideation, be open to these new tangents and pathways.

Cancer Considerations

Seek opportunities for spontaneity
How can you make your medical appointments feel new, incorporating elements of spontaneity? It could be small things like bringing a new friend or parking further away and enjoying a longer walk into the center. Or it could be a little more involved like bringing a small gift of appreciation to a hospital employee like the coffee shop barista, the custodian cleaning the hallways, or your infusion nurse. This unexpected moment of connection will make their day and give you a boost too. Whatever ideas you come up with, remind yourself that keeping things fresh and new will increase your energy.

Question your care team
Challenge your care team by asking for innovative options or ideas that will aid in a smoother treatment, healing, recovery, and survivorship process. You may be curious about integrative care combined with conventional cancer therapies like chemotherapy, radiation, and surgery. Share your curiosities and questions with your care team around nutrition, exercise, relaxation, and stress reduction options. Encourage them to be creative, as you are open to possibilities beyond the status quo.

Plan to combat the boredom
Your creative mind can get easily bored. The healthcare system involves policies, procedures, forms, and waiting. These are less than thrilling for someone like you who thrives on innovation and creativity. Anticipate these bland experiences and strategize ways you'd like to liven them up. This may include the people you bring to appointments, tuning into a new book or podcast while you wait, or purposefully engaging with people you encounter that day.

Create as you wait
Many people with the strength of Ideation are creative. Creativity can take endless forms, so it is impossible to list them all, but you may have

musical, artistic, dance, or writing interests and talents. Could you create something to remember your cancer experience by like a poem, a painting, a clever mantra, or a song? Or maybe you want to channel your creative energy in a direction to distract from your cancer experience. You may want to engage in a new hobby, such as knitting or drawing, to serve as a reprieve from all things cancer. Whatever those interests and talents of yours are, try to do more of them when your energy allows.

Catherine, a cancer survivor in Calgary whose top strength is Ideation shared, "I did not let myself become consumed with attending medical appointments but rather sought out other activities that made my heart happy. There were so many available day programs locally that I tapped into facilitated activities and there were others I discovered on my own. I never had a dull day and used my Ideation strength to come up with ideas on how to best manage each day. This ensured I continued to live a meaningful, joyful existence, so much so that many friends were surprised when I shared that I was going through a cancer journey."

Can you reframe the challenge?

Can you think outside the box regarding the impact cancer will have on your life? Are there ways to reframe the current obstacles? For example, your treatment may cause your hair to fall out, impact the style of clothes you can comfortably wear, or lead you to need walking support. Is there a way to get creative with your new appearance? Some people experiment with new short hairstyles, wigs, hats, or unique outfits. Other survivors may need a cane, walker, or wheelchair for weak muscles or mobility issues. Would you enjoy a walking device decorated with ribbons, your favorite colors, or customized for your personality? Izzy Wheels is a company in Ireland founded by sisters Ailbhe and Izzy Keane that creates unique wheel covers for wheelchairs users.[47] Their vision statement explains, "We want to show the world that wheelchairs can be so much more than a medical device; they can be a piece of artistic self-expression." They have partnered with over 100 artists around the globe

---

47 Izzy Wheels, Wheelchair Wheel Covers: https://www.izzywheels.com.

and brands like Disney, Barbie, and Marvel. Their slogan is "If you can't stand up, stand out™!" How cool is that!?! If any of these creative ideas sound like fun and you will feel some inspiration through experimentation, go for it.

Create a space for your health-related ideating

Think about where you do your best thinking and who might be a great thinking partner to kick ideas around with. Consider going to your favorite thinking spaces, like your screened-in patio or community library, for your health-related ideating. It is important to give yourself time, and arguably extra time, for dreaming and brainstorming. Run your ideas by other cancer survivors or your supporters. Invite them in on the brainstorming process around where to pursue treatment, what path to take, or how to best rest and recover. You'll love the energy this process creates, and their ideas or questions will fuel your creative mind as you work to find the best option for you.

Cancer Cautions

Not all ideas are good ideas

In brainstorming sessions, a common ground rule set up front is "There are no bad ideas." The intent is to free people up to comfortably share whatever comes to their mind, even if it sounds like a wild option. This creates spaces for openness, sharing, vulnerability, and expanded thinking. Those are all great things, and you can still take a brainstorming approach to different aspects of your cancer experience. However, there are bad ideas when it comes to cancer treatment, and research studies can back this statement. So, before you move forward with an idea that came from the philosophy of No Bad Ideas, make sure you run it by an accredited professional who has the expertise to objectively evaluate your decisions.

Your treatment plan does not have to be innovative
Just because you may gravitate toward new and innovative ways of doing things does not mean your treatment plan needs to fall under those categories. If your care team recommends a path that delivers successful outcomes and you feel confident in the plan, you can always incorporate innovation into other aspects of your life.

Includer

People exceptionally talented in the Includer theme accept others. They are instinctively aware of those who feel left out and make an effort to include them.

I had a lot of feelings of my body failing me. I had to work very hard at accepting my body as my partner in fighting cancer, not my enemy. I had to think of my body as a friend that I would give grace to.

—Josie, breast cancer survivor

"Stretch the circle wider." This is your philosophy. As an instinctively accepting person, you hate the idea of someone being ignored or on the outside looking in. You want to include people and make them feel like they are part of the group. While some are drawn to exclusive clubs or cliques, you avoid groups that prohibit some people from joining. You welcome what people have to say without judgment regardless of their status, race, sex, nationality, or faith. Your kindness and inclusive nature are rooted in the belief that people should respect differences and that fundamentally, we all have value and deserve to be included.

Characteristics of Those with Includer Talents

Accepting Interactive Others-sensitive
Sensitive Tolerant Perceptive
Welcoming Integrating

Cancer Connection

You are naturally an open-minded, accepting, and warm person. You see people who are left out or on the fringe when many others don't notice their exclusion. As you go through your cancer experience, who are the people you want to invite in or ensure do not feel left out? Consider the question from the angle of who you want to tell about your diagnosis and health updates. Also, take some time to think about this question and how it applies to medical care team members, perhaps in the form of second and third opinions or referrals to specialists.

Some cancer survivors report feeling betrayed or abandoned by their body when they receive their diagnosis. One survivor, Josie, shared, "I had a lot of feelings of my body failing me. I was a deliberately healthy person, and many people were shocked that even I could get cancer. I had to work very hard at accepting my body as my partner in fighting cancer, not my enemy. I had to think of my body as a friend that I would give grace to." There aren't opposites of strengths, but an opposite of inclusion is exclusion, and it captures the sense that some survivors feel. There can be a feeling of mistrust, anger, and disappointment in your body, and these emotions can get especially complex if your type of cancer leads to removal or altering of body parts. These are real emotions and not to be dismissed, but perhaps, you could make an intentional effort to apply your strength of Includer and show your body more acceptance and less judgment. It can certainly be an ongoing challenge that takes many survivors months, if not years, to achieve.

Cancer Considerations

Ensure all your providers are on the same page
You will consider all providers as part of your care team. Ensure everyone is receiving your medical updates, as appropriate, so you are getting comprehensive, collaborative care. This is typically the standard of care, but it will be especially important to you as you want to ensure all your providers are on the same page. For example, direct your cancer care team to share your medical record updates electronically with your general practitioner.

Who should join you on the journey?
Who would you like to include during your cancer experience? Who is on the guest list and who doesn't make the cut? Your motto may be *The more, the merrier!* but it doesn't have to be true for your cancer experience. In general, the more people you invite to join you, whether physically on appointments or mentally through updates, the more energy you will expend communicating and responding. Check in with yourself about what level of energy and giving feels sustainable to you.

Have backup plans for when you miss out
As you are going through your cancer experience, there may be treatment side effects, fatigue, or simply mental overwhelm and exhaustion. In some situations, this physical or emotional toll could eliminate you from attending events, holiday gatherings, or celebrations with family and friends. This feels extraordinarily difficult for somebody with the strength of Includer. Consider having a few backup plans in mind for if that scenario happens. Are there other cancer survivors or a support group you could reach out to for encouragement? Could you designate somebody to call when you're discouraged that your health is taking you out of a group setting? Let that person know in advance, "When I call you in these situations, I'm feeling really left out." Make sure this is somebody who gets you and is sensitive to that need of yours.

Look forward to helping reduce barriers to care
Given your eye for equality and inclusion, you may quickly notice disparities in healthcare. Take note of the questions you have and the challenges you observe. When you feel up to it, consider how you can help close any gaps in care you've seen. Talk with your oncologist about what donations would help patients, like canned foods or gas gift cards. Ask them about committees or organizations that help cancer survivors facing barriers to care such as financial, transportation, or lack of support. Some cancer survivors serve as patient advocates to help share the patient perspective in the medical community for anything from process improvement to research studies. Arrange a meeting with an elected government official or nonprofit group working to improve health disparities. Voice your concerns and see how you or others can be motivated to help.

Cancer Cautions

Less is sometimes more
You do not need to include everyone in your family or wider circle in your decision-making process. There are other ways to include people who care about you in your cancer experience that would be more rewarding for them and more beneficial to you.

Monitor your health as you learn more about disparities
Depending on where you receive your medical care, you may quickly realize that cancer care is not equally available to all patients depending on a variety of circumstances, such as insurance benefits or geographical constraints in rural areas. You have an eye for when people are being left out and the more you observe and learn about health disparities, this may leave you feeling discouraged or depressed. Your health is your top priority right now, but if you enjoy learning about access to care and looking for areas to help, consider doing so after you conclude treatment or on the days your energy allows.

Individualization

People exceptionally talented in the Individualization theme are intrigued with the unique qualities of each person. They have a gift for figuring out how different people can work together productively.

As I listened carefully to multiple survivors, I was able to tune into their uniqueness and carefully select pieces of their thought processes and experiences that were helpful for customizing my own plan.

—*Barb, breast cancer survivor*

You are intrigued by the unique qualities of each person. Generalizations and stereotypes frustrate you because they obscure people's distinct characteristics. You instinctively focus on the differences between individuals. You want to understand people and figure out why they do what they do. You observe each person's style, motivation, how they think, and how they build relationships because you are fascinated with the cause and effect of human behavior. Your Individualization explains why you pick just the right birthday gift for your friends and why you know that one person prefers praise in public while another detests it. As a keen observer of people, you know how to draw out the best in everyone. While some search for the perfect team structure or process, you know that the secret to a productive team is everyone using their unique strengths to do what they do best every day.

Characteristics of Those with Individualization Talents

Aware	Perceptive	Strengths-oriented	Fair
Insightful	Unique	People-oriented	Astute
Accurate	Diverse		

Cancer Connection

You naturally see the uniqueness in people and are interested in how we each "tick" a little differently. Carry this talent with you as a cancer survivor as you will meet lots of new people from the day of your diagnosis. Some encounters may be brief like a one-off meeting with a genetic counselor or receiving a weekly dose of chemotherapy in a large infusion center from a nurse you may never see again. Other interactions will be repeated, like visits with your oncologist that may extend for many years. Regardless of the length of these relationships, they are all opportunities for you to display your curiosity and learn more about their personal stories. Learning about the caring healthcare professionals you meet will help you bring out the best in your care team and keep you engaged.

You may have a knack for aligning people to specific roles or activities, like a recruiter or talent agent. People want so badly to help you during your cancer experience. If you are fortunate to have supporters nearby, be prepared to receive a pan or two of lasagna or other tangible offers of help. If people ask you, "What can I do to help," use your Individualization strength to steer them in the right direction. I distinctly remember a conversation with our awesome next-door neighbors, Gil and Kris, shortly after receiving my diagnosis. When this conversation came up, Kris offered to cook us a meal, but she made a face indicating that cooking might not be her favorite thing to do and a joke that we might not want to eat what she would make. It was so clear to me in that moment that supporters should play to their strengths, too. In fact, Kris did just that by sending me inspirational quotes and setting flowers on my home office desk as a surprise one day, complete with a metal sign which read "Where there is struggle, there is also strength." It was absolutely perfect! Those gifts from Kris meant so much more to me coming directly from her heart than any pan of lasagna ever could have. While I was so appreciative of the kindness and support from family and friends, I didn't want to put anybody out or have them do something out of obligation. I only wanted them to help where and how they felt most comfortable. Keep that in mind when asking for help and steering your support team.

Although a cancer experience is often challenging and exhausting, this strength will find pockets of goodness along the way through your interactions with people. Your innate interest in people will be fed by your encounters with your care team, meeting other cancer survivors, and building even closer connections with your supporters. Those new and deeper relationships are two of the positive things that I experienced from having cancer.

Cancer Considerations

Get curious about your medical team
Read their bios online and ask them questions about what brought them to their work. They will feel honored to be seen so clearly, and you will get a kick out of learning more about these new and important people in your life. Individualization is my top strength. When I read online that my oncologist graduated from a high school in Olathe, Kansas, less than a mile from where we lived for 10 years, that was an instant connection for us. It was a nice starting point to learn more about Dr. Phadke's path that brought her to Iowa and her current role of teaching and practicing medicine.

Ask what makes your cancer unique
Depending on your cancer, you may quickly realize that there are differences between the same kinds of cancer. For example, prior to my

diagnosis, I thought all breast cancers were the same. I didn't know there are different subtypes of disease, such as hormone positive or triple negative. The subtype of the disease, among other factors, influences the type of treatment plan recommended such as different types of chemotherapy and medications. What works for one subtype of breast cancer does not work for other subtypes. Ask your care team what makes your specific subtype of cancer unique or similar to others. As somebody intrigued by people's uniqueness, you will find that medical conversation fascinating.

Match the strengths of your supporters to your needs

You are exceptionally good at seeing people's talents and skills. You innately know that we are all unique, and you can see how a person's strengths can be used in a role or as part of a team. If your family, friends, colleagues, or other supporters are asking you what they can do to help, take your time to think about each person's strengths before responding. Some may be the perfect people to join you for a morning walk outside, others may be excellent cooks and offer a home-cooked meal, and some may be perfect for a behind-the-scenes researching role looking up a certain article or product that you'd like to learn more about. As people offer to help, don't hesitate to make specific requests based on the strengths you see in them. They will love the opportunity to support you in an area where they shine.

During my cancer experience, there was one hot summer day in July where I was extremely fatigued and nauseated. My good friend and golfing partner, Lori, was planning to stop by and chat that afternoon. Lori is an excellent communicator. In fact, Communication is one of her top strengths and she works at a local university as an advising coordinator and instructor in the department of communication and media. I would have canceled nearly any other obligation that day, but I knew that a visit from Lori would boost my nearly empty gas tank. I was right. She brought me a healthy green smoothie and we had a great time chatting together. Use your knowledge of other peoples' strengths to your advantage to help give you a boost when you need it most.

Consider multiple perspectives

You value diversity and have probably always been curious about people. That may have contributed to your life in the role of counselor, observer, listener, or partner among others. Use this open mindset to connect with cancer survivors, supporters, or even care providers to consider multiple perspectives, ideas, and opinions. While other cancer survivors may be overwhelmed by the varying ideas and recommendations, you will be able to remain objective since you naturally understand where they are coming from.

Barb has the strength of Individualization and shared:

> It was helpful for me to hear about the plan other breast cancer survivors followed and what drove them to make those decisions. I evaluated those insights to help me come to the treatment decision that was best for me. As I listened carefully to the decision-making processes of multiple survivors, I was able to tune into their uniqueness and carefully select pieces of their thought processes and experiences that were helpful for customizing my own plan.

Customize your communications

You are a customizer. You may naturally create plans for how you share your diagnosis differently, depending on your audience. One cancer survivor shared, "I customized my communications plan. My group of friends called the October Girls would get a different email than other groups of people." This helped her share the same health information in a different style and packaging depending on who was opening the message in their inbox.

Volunteer or advocate

Consider using your people-oriented approach as a volunteer for a non-profit cancer organization or an advocate in the political arena. These opportunities expose you to a wide variety of personalities and many people, who may bring diverse perspectives, yet are similarly passionate about making improvements in the cancer arena.

Cancer Cautions

You may not be seen as unique
Be prepared for some parts of your medical experience to feel generic and standardized. Although you naturally see each person as a unique individual, you may not have that approach reciprocated by all medical professionals or processes. For example, check-in procedures are close to identical for Cancer Patient 1 as they are for Cancer Patient 2. You stand at the counter, state your name and date of birth, and the registration clerk enters information into the computer and hands you a tablet to complete your online registration. There are certainly good reasons for this to be a uniform, efficient process. Just be prepared that you may not feel uniquely seen during some portions of your visits.

Give people the benefit of the doubt
Some people may show their support by sharing the experiences of other cancer survivors. They may say things like "My aunt had a bone marrow transplant too," or "When my boss went through chemo, he was so sick and could barely work." Although their motivation may be to connect with you on such a personal topic, it can sometimes land awkwardly or just be wrong.

Try to give people the benefit of the doubt that they mean well and may be nervous or unsure what to say. If that doesn't help, you can let them know that every cancer survivor is unique, and you are doing your best to focus on your own experience versus those of other people.

Input

People exceptionally talented in the Input theme have a need to collect and archive. They may accumulate information, ideas, artifacts, or even relationships.

> I wanted the binder to feel uplifting to me. It went with me to every appointment, giving me places to put all the reports and information I was given. It helped on a practical and emotional level.
>
> —Mary Sue, breast cancer survivor

You are inquisitive. You collect things. You might collect information—facts, books, or quotations—or you might collect tangible objects. Whatever it is, you collect it because it interests you. And you find so many things interesting. The world is exciting because of its infinite variety and complexity. When you read, it is not necessarily to refine your theories, but to add information to your archives. When you travel, each new location offers new souvenirs and facts that you can acquire and store away. Why are they worth saving? You might not know exactly when or why you will need them, but with so many possible uses, you don't feel comfortable throwing anything away. So you keep acquiring and compiling. It keeps your mind fresh. Perhaps one day, some of it will be valuable.

Characteristics of Those with Input Talents

Resourceful   Inquisitive   Generous
Knowledgeable   Collecting   Utility-aware
Well-read   Investigative

Cancer Connection

Receiving a cancer diagnosis is often accompanied by information overload but not for you. People with Input as a strength are typically armed with resources, knowledge, and tools. You excel at learning more about a subject and collecting info. You will be bombarded with details about your diagnosis, potential treatment plans, timelines, and various resources. There are so many ideas, questions, and opinions coming your way from medical professionals, family members, friends, and your research. Keep in mind that you are naturally inquisitive and skilled in gathering tools and information. That's a real advantage right now so let yourself lean on your collecting and gathering instincts.

The key to making this strength valuable is using the available information and tools versus having it. Simply researching healthcare institutions and providers doesn't start the motor on your cancer treatment. My Strengths teacher, Curt Liesveld, shared this great example on Gallup's *Theme Thursday* podcast.

> The metaphor I often use with this theme is a sponge. Just like a sponge is absorbent, people with Input can absorb stuff. Now I tell people, the purpose of a sponge is never to be a permanent container. In fact, when a sponge holds on to stuff a little too long it starts to smell a bit. A sponge is really a dispenser or transporter from one place to another, and I think the core value of people with Input is their resourcefulness.[48]

---

[48] Gallup CliftonStrengths. "Input: Learning to Love All 34 Talent Themes." Available at: https://www.gallup.com/cliftonstrengths/en/251180/input-learning-love-talent-themes.aspx.

You have to take action with the information you've gathered to start your healing. One cancer survivor shared that she "took agency and got myself as equipped as I could" by gathering credible information from comprehensive cancer centers.

Mary Sue Ingraham, a breast cancer survivor with the Input strength shared:

> Once it looked like there was a good chance I had a malignancy, I felt a sense of overwhelm. I realized that collecting all the relevant information and reports would not only be practical and help me stay organized but also would help allay my sense of being overwhelmed. I put together a binder with dividers for all the categories of information that would be coming—lab and diagnostic results, notes from visits with physicians, and contact information for providers. I wanted the binder to feel uplifting to me, so I got one with a transparent cover over the front and put a beautiful photograph of a rushing mountain river in it. That binder went with me to every appointment, giving me places to put all the various reports and information I was given. It helped on a practical and emotional level.

You'll have the opportunity to not only gather information, but also tools and products that will help improve your experiences with treatment. Due to your knack for investigating options, either from materials you read or people you speak with, you'll know the best ways to prepare for major phases of your treatment plan. You understand that useful information is available, and you may approach finding it like a quest or a scavenger hunt. This willingness to dig and explore means you'll gain more ideas and perspectives than many survivors. Even if what you uncover isn't a product or path you decide to pursue, the act of exploring additional information will help you feel more confident in your care decisions. When you are ready, you can share what you've gathered to help other cancer survivors and caregivers get a head start. As Curt recommends, don't hold onto that information forever.

Cancer Considerations

Create an information storage plan

Create a system to organize and easily access the health information you gather. Remember it's about *using* the information, so you don't need to research all the ways to organize health information, and your system doesn't need to be perfect. Make sure you have a place for physical resources like books and journals, printed medical results, and handouts from your care team. If possible, take this step early in your diagnosis. In addition to a physical location for storage of items, create electronic systems like Notes files on your phone, a designated folder within your email, and shortcuts on your web browser for websites you visit frequently. You can also use an electronic notebook like Evernote or Notion. You'll also receive recommendations like cancer survivors to speak to, cancer centers, physicians, healthcare providers, diet and supplement suggestions. By creating a reliable storage structure, you will have confidence that all the resources you're collecting will be easily found when you need them. Jen, a mucosal melanoma cancer survivor with Input, shared that she could never imagine getting rid of her freckle binder!

Define enough

Get clear on the purpose of your knowledge gathering and define what will be enough for you. This will help you sift through the masses of information and advice available, saving you time and stress. For example, when will you have enough information to decide what to bring for your first chemotherapy appointment or your overnight stay in the hospital for surgery? Do you need to read responses from more than 25 people in a private Facebook group from your care center? Or maybe you are comfortable talking with one or two cancer survivors and letting their insights be enough to inform your packing strategy. Challenge yourself to ask, "Will one more piece of information on this topic change my decision or path forward?" If not, you may not need to keep digging or asking questions. Additionally, you may learn some information that you won't need until later. For example, your diagnosis may call for surgery followed by chemotherapy. As you're talking with survivors about their surgery process and questions you have, they may also share insights about chemotherapy. Save that information for the future.

Control your research time

Consider how to incorporate adding time limits and structure to your gathering process. You may set timers and alarms for how long you're willing to spend researching a topic like the best skin creams for radiation burns. If you'd like to talk with other colon cancer survivors about how they cared for their incisions and drains after their colon resection, decide how many experiences you need to hear to feel prepared. Instead of talking with six survivors, you may feel like you know enough to feel confident for your surgery after one conversation. Remind yourself that just because you have access to lots of resources, you may not need to exhaust all of them.

Delegate what you can

What research can you delegate? You are still the decision-maker, but would it be helpful to have others begin the information gathering process for you? Your supporters could get the process started by exploring where to buy a wig, or whether insurance covers a certain medical product, or finding out local support group meeting times.

If you feel that two items need to be explored simultaneously, ask for help with the one that is lower in priority, or the item further out on the horizon. For example, you may be considering two different cancer centers and spending significant time evaluating those options. At both institutions, surgery may be your first step and you feel unprepared or uninformed about the procedure. As you prioritize selecting the best care team for your needs, consider delegating the surgery research to a trusted supporter. Once you have bandwidth to switch gears and learn about the surgery, they can at least point you in the right direction to begin your learning.

Let something meaningful bring you joy

Do you have a favorite cancer souvenir or keepsake? Is there something that brings you inspiration or joy on the journey? It could be a special card, quote, bracelet, blanket, or a pair of socks somebody gave you as a gift. Put this someplace where you can see and enjoy it. This souvenir could inspire you for years.

You could be a resource for other cancer survivors

You are an amazing resource to other people and have probably already shared countless ideas, articles, data, files, and connections with friends, colleagues, and family over the years. You will approach your new cancer diagnosis with the same inquisitiveness and be a great resource for other cancer survivors if that is a role of interest. Even though there is so much cancer information available online, there is nothing quite like hearing from somebody who has actually experienced the disease. It's the difference between book smarts and street smarts. If sharing cancer-related information, experiences, and advice with others is of interest to you, consider capturing notes of your lessons learned along the way. The opportunities to give back to the cancer community are endless. Think of this like materials you would have collected for a wedding, open house, camping trip, or tailgate party. You have saved a ready-to-unpack-and-use bundle of information, supplies, and other helpful tools. Think about who can benefit from your cancer-related bundle. Depending on your interests, skills, and other strengths, you may be an excellent writer, speaker, mentor, or patient advocate. Opportunities are also available to serve on cancer-related nonprofit boards or committees. Your willingness to share ideas and resources will be highly valued in these groups. It's powerful hearing directly from cancer survivors who have walked the walk.

Christine Carpenter is a great example of a cancer survivor putting her Input strength into motion. She was diagnosed with breast cancer in 1993 and she quickly dug into all the books, resources, and information available. Because of advice she read, Christine joined the National Breast Cancer Coalition and has been the Iowa Field Coordinator for over 30 years. She has spent decades traipsing across the state, meeting with senators and representatives as well as political candidates. I've witnessed Christine's relentless approach in the halls of Congress and have been blown away by the passion, commitment, and knowledge she puts toward ending breast cancer.

Monitor your energy

Pay close attention to the impact of absorbing cancer information on your mood, energy, and sleep patterns. Are you energized after talking with other survivors and reading about cancer, or does it evoke fear, anxiety, uncertainty, and confusion? If you feel energized, this process is likely beneficial for you to feel confident about the decisions you're making about your treatment and care. If it's the latter, you should request a referral to a psychologist, therapist, or support group to manage these feelings. Additionally, what may begin as invigorating and power-generating may hit a tipping point. Picture filling a vase with water before adding a beautiful bouquet of flowers. Water is life-giving to your flowers, yet the vase can only hold so much of it. While you may flourish with the information you initially uncover, be prepared for the law of diminishing returns to strike. At a certain point, more and more information about the same topic or question may no longer add value. Know when enough is enough and be ready to move on to an action, a decision, or next steps.

Cancer Cautions

Beware of bad information

Remember that not all information is created equally. Some information you discover will be misleading, inaccurate, or wrong. Be extremely cautious of what resources you're consuming online. Jen shared, "Your doctor saying, 'Stay off Google!' was nice but not real." I agree with Jen and would not take this advice literally as there are incredible support groups, survivor pages, and practical tips available online. But I might add, "Stay off Google without a direction, credibility filter, and time limit." You want to ensure you know what type of information you're specifically seeking, what accredited institutions or qualified cancer specialists you'll listen to, and how much time you'll allow yourself to surf. Just as you can find pretty rotten recipes for soups and cakes online, you can find some pretty scary, inaccurate, and non-credible cancer advice too.

Rely on the experts
You are likely not a cancer expert unless that is your field of work. You do not need to become a cancer expert. Although you'll naturally want to dig into information and resources, you do not have to find all the answers. Do not let your lack of knowledge in this arena frustrate you. There are experts who have been studying cancer for decades. Surround yourself with an exceptional care team and ask them to direct you to the best resources. Their insight will provide you with a much better place to start than a simple online search or trip to the library. Release the pressure of feeling like you need to gather all the information yourself. Use your resources wisely to help your information gathering process be more efficient, productive, and accurate, and less stressful.

Review and trim away the excess
Beware of information overload and be prepared to recognize when you've hit your limit. If you find yourself swimming in too many links, names, and books, and too much data, you may need to rein in your information gathering or, at a minimum, take a break from it. While knowledge is power, be cautious of overthinking and overanalyzing. Challenge yourself by asking, "What information can I release?" There may be pictures on your phone, articles collected from your oncologist, or books from the library. If these things evoke ideas or fears about cancer that aren't serving you now and likely won't in the future, it's time for them to receive the delete button, land in the recycle bin, or slide down the library return box. If you are stuck in a cycle of paralysis by analysis and delaying forward movement, ask yourself, "What information do I need to take the next step forward?" If you still feel frozen, reach out to your support team and medical professionals to revisit the information and options.

Intellection

People exceptionally talented in the Intellection theme enjoy deep thinking. They are introspective and appreciate intellectual discussions.

After years of being told I was incurable, I was declared cancer-free. But there's no going back. I am forever changed by what I discovered: *life is so beautiful and life is so hard. For everyone.*

—Dr. Kate Bowler, Professor of Religious History at Duke University and colon cancer survivor

You like to think. You like exercising the "muscles" of your brain, stretching them in multiple directions. Your need for mental activity may be focused. For example, you might be trying to solve a problem, develop an idea, or understand another person's actions. Sometimes, you may think about practical matters such as the events of the day or a conversation you plan to have. The exact focus will depend on your other strengths. There might be times when your mental activity lacks focus. Intellection does not dictate what you think about, just that you like to think. You are introspective, and you enjoy time alone to reflect. You are your own best companion as you ask yourself questions and experiment with answers to see how they sound. This musing will always be a natural part of your life.

Characteristics of Those with Intellection Talents

Introspective	Intellectual	In-depth	Discontented
Intense	Driven	Solitary	Philosophical
Reflective	Thinking	Musing	

Cancer Connection

Receiving a cancer diagnosis and experiencing treatment is a very reflective time for most people—there is so much to think about. Because of your Intellection strength you may find yourself doing a lot of deep thinking. Your serious and thoughtful approach will suit you as you navigate your cancer diagnosis. Although you will probably feel a sense of urgency to move your treatment forward quickly, remind yourself that you are at your best when you have time to think deeply. When faced with challenging situations in the past, giving yourself that buffer of time has allowed you to feel calmer and more confident about your choices. Ask your cancer team about the ideal timeline for your treatment decisions. For example, one surgeon told me when I received my diagnosis in May that I could take time to consider my options, but he added, "Don't wait all summer." This let me know that a few days would not impact my outcomes, but waiting a few months was not recommended. Once you understand that window, claim that buffer of time for analyzing and processing your options if it is safe to do so.

Information is the food of Intellection so you may have more questions than other cancer survivors. Don't hesitate to gather all the information you need to feed your thoughts. This will aid in better decision-making.

Clarity is a critical word for you to remember as people with the strength of Intellection are known for gaining clarity or sharing it with others after they've spent time thinking, typically alone. What circumstances have led to clarity for you in the past? Is there a certain time of day, location, or process that sets you up for your best thinking? If there are people you enjoy engaging in deep discussions or debates, bring them into your circle. Purposely work to recreate these settings frequently to allow yourself the ideal environment for reflection. This intentionality will pay off in increased calmness, confidence, and clarity as you move forward with your cancer experience.

Cancer Considerations

Give yourself the gift of downtime
People with the strength of Intellection tend to have better ideas, strategies, and suggestions with time. You may enjoy a little downtime, me-time, or windshield time while driving in the car. This may look like needing time to process your diagnosis before sharing it with others. It could include clarifying timelines with your care team and seeing if you can take a few hours, days, or weeks before making treatment decisions. One cancer survivor suggested taking a day off from new information and allowing yourself some downtime. She shared, "There was a whirlwind of activity going on, and I hit a point where I couldn't take in any more information. I needed to sit and digest this first." Although you may prefer a supporting role over the lead part, people will be looking to you to understand what you are going through, and what you need. If you feel overwhelmed with their questions, you can always say, "Can I think about that and get back to you?" Don't hesitate to enlist your thinking partners as you work through these important decisions.

Set your roster and guard your time
Now is the time for you to share your preferences about who joins you for different aspects of your cancer experience. If you welcome friends or family to attend doctor's appointments with you, invite them along. If you'd rather go alone or with one other person, great. People will be paying closer attention to you than normal. You likely talk less than many of your friends and family members. Invite them to join you for

appointments if you think it will be comforting to have them around to create small talk, distract you, or to lift your spirits. Express your desire for downtime if you reach a point where you'd prefer to sleep, read, or zone out. Everyone will be happy to create the best environment for your health and healing, even if it means respecting your desire for solitude.

In your life prior to cancer, did you get enough alone time? People with Intellection need time to think alone. If you typically felt overwhelmed and drained from too much social interaction, your cancer diagnosis may provide an opportunity for you to create more boundaries on your time. Although your diagnosis may increase the number of interactions from concerned friends and family, it can also provide you with great justification for additional alone time. This could look like earlier bedtimes, fewer social engagements, working from home, and canceling volunteer commitments. Your desire to recharge your batteries by being alone or in a small group should always be honored but may sometimes feel ignored by your extroverted friends and family members who just want to help. They'll get over it. Be clear with your requests to get what you need to heal.

Seek quality conversations
Are there people in your life who you enjoy engaging in deep, thought-provoking conversations? Consider reaching out to them to discuss topics around cancer, health, or life in general. Arrange time to meet for coffee, spend time together on a video conference, or email or text with them. Their thoughtful insights will fuel your need for reflection and debate. This bantering process of exchanging deep thoughts will boost your energy and fuel your mind.

Share your wisdom
What have you been thinking about that others need to hear? Given your introspective nature, you will continue to do plenty of deep thinking, potentially on new topics. Who needs to understand your new thoughts, ideas, or decisions related to your cancer, health, schedule, requests, or needs for support? If sharing your inner dialog with a colleague, counselor,

physician, friend, or loved one would be beneficial for your health, push yourself to get it out of your head and into the open for others to discuss and help you. According to Gallup's *Theme Thursday* podcast, *Intellection: Learning to Love All 34 Talent Themes*,[49] the challenge that people with Intellection have is that "Your wisdom and understanding is wasted if it remains in your head. Somehow it needs to get out of your mouth or through your pen." Do this in service to yourself and perhaps, other cancer patients.

Write

If you have thoughts and words that need to go somewhere, but you're not ready to share with somebody you know, pick up a pen or fire up your computer. It's time to start writing. People with the strength of Intellection are often incredible writers. Don't put any pressure on yourself that your work needs to be published. It may never see the light of day, but the act of getting these thoughts out of your head will give you a productive mood boost. Your words may live privately in a notebook, a journal, on a computer screen, or publicly on social media, a blog, or a community support page. Wherever your words travel, be sure that the process of writing provides positive energy for you and not a source of stress or perfectionism.

Cancer Cautions

Beware of rumination

Although you enjoy spending time alone with your thoughts, action is also necessary. Assess your cancer and health-related thoughts frequently. Ask yourself, "Is this just a fleeting thought, theory, or idea, or is this something I need to put into action?" While having an active mind is not new to you, be aware if you are trending toward rumination, that is,

---

49 Gallup's *Theme Thursday* podcast, "Intellection: Learning to Love All 34 Talent Themes." Available at: https://www.gallup.com/cliftonstrengths/en/251228/intellection-learning-love-talent-themes.aspx.

"obsessional thinking involving excessive, repetitive thoughts or themes that interfere with other forms of mental activity,"[50] especially around your diagnosis and future. Pay attention to how your thoughts make you feel and reach out to a member of your care team, a counselor, psychologist, or support group if you sense they are interfering with your daily life and your ability to take care of yourself.

Many forms of cancer need to be treated quickly. Although you will rarely, if ever, need to make a medical decision on the spot, you do need to be prepared to take action. Get informed, gather resources, ask questions, and work to make timely decisions. Engage someone you trust in your decision-making process if timeliness is crucial. Do not delay decisions that could negatively impact your health outcomes and be prepared to channel your thoughtful questions into actions.

You may not find comfort in clichés

Not everyone shares your desire for nuanced, intellectual viewpoints and looking at all sides of a question. You know that cancer is a complex, sophisticated disease and can't be boiled down to generic clichés. Words that are meant to provide you comfort and relief may annoy you. People may say things like *you're so strong*, or *everything happens for a reason*, or *screw cancer*. If sayings like these irritate or upset you, it's fine to let that person know you would rather not talk about your cancer. Keep in mind the intent behind people's words and that they are likely coming from a place of support and caring. On that note, I loved reading Dr. Kate Bowler's New York Times bestseller, *Everything Happens for a Reason: And Other Lies I've Loved*.[51] When she was just 35, the young mother and professor of religious history at Duke University was diagnosed with Stage 4 colon cancer with chances of survival about one in ten. Dr. Bowler endured years of grueling treatment and this book "tells her story, offering up her irreverent, hard-won observations on dying and the ways it has taught her to live." She says, "After years of being told I

---

50 APA Dictionary of Psychology: https://dictionary.apa.org/rumination.
51 Bowler, Kate. https://katebowler.com.

was incurable, I was declared cancer-free. But there's no going back. I am forever changed by what I discovered: Life is so beautiful and life is so hard. For everyone."

Learner

People exceptionally talented in the Learner theme have a great desire to learn and want to continuously improve. The process of learning, rather than the outcome, excites them.

You love to learn. The subjects that interest you most will depend on your other themes and experiences, but you will always be drawn to learning. The process of learning, more than the content or the result, is especially exciting for you. The steady progression from ignorance to competence energizes you—the thrill of the first few facts, the early efforts to recite or practice what you have learned, the growing confidence of a skill mastered. You love to engage in new experiences. For example, exploring new activities or fields of study might energize you. You thrive in dynamic environments where you can learn a lot about a new subject in a short period of time and then move on. You do not necessarily want to become the subject matter expert or earn a professional or academic credential. For you, the outcome is less significant than the journey.

I used what I learned in school to do cancer better. I researched surgeries, doctors, and medicines, of course, but I'm also educating myself on recovering better.

—Josie, PhD nursing student and breast cancer survivor

Characteristics of Those with Learner Talents

Curious	Inquisitive	Studious
Competent	Interested	Open-minded
Passionate		

Cancer Connection

People with the strength of Learner love new experiences, growth opportunities, and uncovering ways to continuously improve. Navigating a cancer diagnosis and treatment plan will leave you no shortage of opportunities to practice learning. Your cancer experience will bring new people, places, and events into your life. These may include a new hospital, clinic, medicine, physician, side effect, or personal connection. Challenge yourself to shift your perspective from fear and worry to curiosity and competency.

You are naturally energized when expanding your perspectives and exploring cutting-edge information and ideas. Learner is one of my Top 5 strengths and one I used often during my treatment and continue to use years later. I asked my oncologist a lot of questions, and she was amazing with her thorough responses and willingness to follow up with even more information. She also has Learner as a top strength, number one to be exact, so our visits were always energizing. As a result of my questions and desire to learn more, Dr. Phadke provided referrals to an oncology psychologist, a holistic physician, and an oncology dietitian. I was also eager to gain new ideas and resources and attended a six-week mindfulness course with other cancer survivors, a local Look Good Feel Better make-up and hair class,[52] and a local cancer survivors support group while bald and exhausted from chemotherapy. I got involved in advocacy efforts and meetings with our state politicians in Washington, D.C., and Des Moines. Adding these

---

52 Look Good Feel Better: https://lookgoodfeelbetter.org.

additional appointments, classes, and resources boosted my energy levels and helped me feel more informed and empowered in an extremely overwhelming time of my life as a young mom.

You find life interesting. You know that there is always more to learn and can get bored if things are stagnant. Cancer will regrettably give you plenty to explore—you will not get bored during this experience. You may take a deep dive learning about your disease, or your curiosity may take you in other personal, professional, or inner-growth directions. Regardless, remember that even small moments of learning give you huge rewards. Although your body will likely be tired from treatment, medications, or stress, your mind will be fueled by the opportunity to develop and grow. Use the awareness of your Learner strength to your advantage as you push to ask questions, seek resources, and remain open to varying perspectives along the way.

Cancer Considerations

Stay curious
Many cancer survivors I've spoken with who have Learner as a strength found certain aspects of the process fascinating. You will too. Pay attention to what you're curious about as you navigate this health situation. How can you learn more about any cancer-related topics of interest such as clinical trials, nutrition, or mindset? That doesn't mean you need to go back to school to become a cancer researcher or oncologist: simply notice what makes you sit up a little taller or get that inner feeling of *I need to know more*. Many cancer survivors with the Learner talent are amazed that their treatment included things that made their path easier, more convenient, less painful, or even life-changing.

Some examples people have shared with me:
- Being fascinated by the Neulasta® on-body injector shot you receive to reduce the risk of infection from strong chemotherapy
- Excitement about joining a clinical trial to aid in medical progress

- Pursuing advanced treatment options such as immunotherapy or CAR T-cell therapy
- Using scalp hypothermia through cold caps to reduce hair loss from chemotherapy
- Undergoing more advanced and sophisticated surgery procedures like DIEP flap
- Benefiting from FDA newly approved life-saving medication that was unavailable even 10 years prior

Treat this as an opportunity for learning

You are energized by fresh, new experiences. Can you mentally position your treatment phases as something new to explore? Let yourself ask probing questions of your medical team, supporters, and other cancer survivors. Your learning curiosity may be geared more toward people, or processes, or products and resources. If you are curious about people, get to know your care team and ask questions about their career paths and desire to study cancer. If you enjoy learning about processes, such as meditation practices, or products such as the chemotherapy drugs, ask about what you're observing or experiencing. Ask for referrals when you'd like to dig deeper with an expert on any of the topics, if necessary. Tap into this opportunity to grow and evolve through your cancer experience.

Does your learning lead to additional action?

You may be intrigued by cancer data, statistics, and research. Or you may seek learning on a completely different subject. You may turn your energy toward your hobbies, such as gardening or cooking, as your energy allows. Or you may dig in on your career path, educational opportunities, or ways to contribute to your community. Wherever you find yourself exploring and growing, do you want to put this knowledge into motion or use it purposefully? Check in with yourself to see if you have an interest in doing anything with all you're learning. It's good to understand if you are learning for the sake of learning or if you are seeing a bigger picture or plan unfolding with this new knowledge. Both options are equally acceptable given that the process of learning invigorates you and increases your energy.

Josie was pursuing her PhD in nursing with an emphasis in health systems when she received her cancer diagnosis. She shared, "I never let cancer be a reason to pause school. I used what I learned in school to do cancer better. I researched surgeries, doctors, and medicines, of course, but I'm also educating myself on recovering better. I'm learning about how to manage side effects and how to decrease my chances of recurrence. I started using red light therapy regularly on my chest and face after chemotherapy sessions. I believe it kept my cell counts up, as evidenced by my labs, so I felt better throughout treatment. It also greatly decreased my pain after my hysterectomy. Another example of leveraging my Learner strength is how I've approached food and nutrition. If I learn about a food or nutrient that has a positive effect on health, I do my research, and then if I decide it's worth trying, I look for a way to incorporate it into my daily salads for lunch. I don't get overwhelmed by the nutritional information; instead, I have fun with prepping salads with all the different colors, nuts, flaxseed, chia seeds, and a good protein. I've noticed that when I skip my salad for lunch, I have more fatigue and joint pain in the days following. I am always looking for correlations between what I eat and how I feel, doing more research, and adjusting based on what I learn."

Share your learnings

Can you do a little teaching during your doctor's appointments? I enjoyed bringing new friends to chemotherapy sessions with me because the whole process was fascinating to me. By sharing that world with friends and loved ones, I gained energy by talking and teaching, and I think they gained energy by being there to support me along the way.

Toward the end of my six months of treatment, close friends asked if I'd be willing to connect with one of their dear friends who had just been diagnosed with breast cancer. We both have Learner as a top strength, and it didn't take too many text messages for me to realize that my conversations with Autumn were going to be more of a roundabout circle drive than a one-way street. Autumn was very similar to me in her growth mindset and eagerness to learn all she could about ways to improve her energy levels and outcomes. Our text threads are filled with links to reputable cancer websites, articles about clinical trials, screenshots, book recommendations, and data points comparing our lab results. We bantered back and forth with questions varying from medications and side effects to nutrition and sunscreen recommendations. I felt much more like a colleague—and sometimes student—of hers than a teacher or mentor. What began as me supporting Cody and Jina's friend quickly evolved into her also supporting me as we learned how to navigate our life detours and cancer survivorship together.

If you enjoy sharing your knowledge, ask your care team for opportunities with local organizations or nonprofits that may be a fit for your desire to teach and support. Other sharing opportunities may include local cancer support groups or volunteering to support those newly diagnosed.

Cancer Cautions

Get clear on your learning goals
Be clear on your learning goals before you begin. Do you need to understand about all forms of a specific cancer, or only yours? Is it helpful or overwhelming for you to understand the history of your type of cancer? Because there is often no limit to the length you'll go to learn about a topic, know that you could find yourself wading through grim information when you are learning about cancer. If your treatment plan and health-related steps are clear and decided, make sure you are not jeopardizing your mental well-being by digging deeper into irrelevant information.

Prioritize what you need to know now
Remind yourself that you won't become a cancer expert overnight unless you are already working in that field. While your inquisitive mind may

want to take a deep dive into all the books, websites, and data, work to prioritize the type of information that you truly need right now. One vaginal melanoma cancer survivor shared, "I thought I could learn my way out of this. That's just who I am. The more I learned, the more questions I had. At some point, I realized that I could trust that people would take care of me even if I didn't have all the answers."

Beware of poor data and suspicious information

Be cautious of misinformation, false claims, frauds, and scams. Your eagerness to learn the latest and greatest around your cancer could lead you to fringe websites or resources. Be vigilant about what you consume. It is usually wise to start with well-known websites created by major medical groups, universities, or well-known advocacy groups. If you find new, interesting, or conflicting information, be sure to share it with your medical team prior to making any decisions.

Maximizer

People exceptionally talented in the Maximizer theme consistently ask, "How can we make this better?" They don't settle for "good enough," but push for excellence.

> Surround yourself with people who help you succeed. There is no doubt that I have overcome so much medical trauma because I have been so lucky to have excellent people around me.
>
> —Laura, Gallup-Certified Strengths Coach and car accident survivor

"Can we make this better?" Excellence, not average, is your standard. For you, taking something from mediocre to good requires a great deal of effort and is not very rewarding. However, transforming something good into something great takes just as much effort but is far more thrilling. Strengths, your own and other people's, fascinate you. You instinctively notice the signs of a potential strength—a glimpse of natural excellence, rapid learning, or a skill mastered. When you see these clues, you are compelled to nurture, refine, and push them toward excellence. You are drawn to others who have cultivated their strengths. Likewise, you prefer to spend time with people who appreciate your unique strengths and avoid those who want to fix you or make you well-rounded. You don't want to waste your life focusing on your weaknesses. You want to capitalize on what you're best at. It's more productive and a lot more fun.

Characteristics of Those with Maximizer Talents

Selective	Quality-oriented	Strengths-obsessed
Discriminating	Judging	Dissatisfied
Strengths-oriented	Results-oriented	Excellence-aware
Choosy	Sorting	

Cancer Connection

You have a desire for quality and an internal drive for excellence. As a cancer survivor, you may push for better answers, better resources, and better overall care. People with Maximizer talents pay attention to strengths—their own and those of others. This natural recognition of talent and potential leads you to want to spend more of your time developing areas where you already have strength rather than only spending time shoring up your weaknesses. This approach to how you spend your time and energy will transfer into how you approach your cancer treatment and survivorship.

Sometimes people with this strength are drawn toward specialists and experts. This may impact where you opt to pursue your medical care. I have Maximizer as a strength, and it impacted how I selected my care team. My breast cancer was the most common subtype called HR+/HER2-.[53] This subtype accounts for 70% of all breast cancers diagnosed and could have been treated locally less than 10 minutes from our house given its common prevalence. Although I considered that option, once I looked at the University of Iowa Health Care (UIHC) website, my decision was made. UIHC's Holden Comprehensive Cancer Center is the only NCI-Designated Cancer Center in Iowa. To date, there are just 72

---

53 National Cancer Institute Cancer Stat Facts: Female Breast Cancer Subtypes: https://seer.cancer.gov/statfacts/html/breast-subtypes.html.

NCI-Designated Cancer Centers in 36 states across the United States.[54] I loved learning that I would get to see a specialist at UIHC, such as a surgeon who only performed breast cancer surgeries, rather than a generalist who may perform a mastectomy in the morning and an appendectomy in the afternoon. While both outcomes may have been identical, I felt comforted knowing I would be in the hands of a specialist at a comprehensive cancer center. If Maximizer wasn't as prominent a talent for me, I might have opted to save time and mileage and receive my treatment locally as many others with similar diagnoses do.

Most people with the strength of Maximizer do not love the common saying, *Sometimes good is good enough*. Although that may be true in many circumstances, most people like you either do not agree with it or don't want to admit that it could be true. Keep this saying in mind on both fronts: If your care is not feeling up to par to you, for whatever reason, express this in the most appropriate way. You know what great looks like, and if you aren't receiving it from a care team member or an institution, share that feedback. On the second front, accept the sentiment and let yourself be okay with *good being enough sometimes*. For example, you may usually like to have a spotless kitchen when you shut the lights off and go upstairs to bed, but fatigue is zapping your energy. Some nights it will be fine to leave a few dishes in the sink and call it good. Remember, sometimes good is good enough—especially when you need to conserve your energy for things you need to make great.

Cancer Considerations

Concentrate on what's going right
Stay focused on strengths. If you have a few side effects or setbacks of your treatment but the overall plan is progressing well, challenge yourself to spend more time talking and thinking about what's going right rather

---

54 NCI-Designated Cancer Centers: https://www.cancer.gov/research/infrastructure/cancer-centers.

than what's going wrong. You are energized by strengths, and this intentional mindset will give you an energy boost.

Help others see their own strengths
Pay attention to the unique talents of your care team members, supporters, caregivers, and those you interact with throughout your treatment. Share what you see. Describe their talents with specific details and compliment them when they deliver great care. You will enjoy talking about their strengths, and they will obviously enjoy validation of their expertise.

Look for ways to replicate your best days
You prefer it when things run smoothly, so pay attention to which appointments go better than others. Does it have something to do with the day of the week, the time of day, what you've had to eat before, who is joining you for the appointment, or another factor? Continue to pay attention to the small details of your appointment and non-appointment days and try to recreate moments from the best days so that you can have more of them in the future.

Keep trying different options
You may really enjoy the process of experimenting with different habits, routines, schedules, or products during your cancer experience. People with Maximizer talents love taking something that is already good and making it even better. Richelle is a Gallup-Certified Strengths Coach based in Colorado whose life changed forever when she was 15 years old. She was out of town for volleyball tryouts and involved in a rollover car accident where she was ejected and had injuries to her back, ribs, pelvis, and hip socket. A Flight for Life® helicopter[55] transported her to Colorado Springs where she had surgery within 12 hours of the accident, yet didn't remember the first of her four months in the hospital. Richelle was initially paralyzed and used a wheelchair for 1½ years before progress-

---

55 CommonSpirit. "Flight for Life." https://www.mountain.commonspirit.org/our-ecosystem/flight-for-life.

ing to a walker, a cane, and other support tools. She was even told she wouldn't be able to carry children. She has two.

As she reflected on the accident and the early years following, Richelle shared, "It never occurred to me to be a permanent situation." She described having to learn how to put socks on despite not being able to feel her legs. She had to navigate a variety of terrain and carefully evaluate different steps, curbs, rocks, and pebbles along the path of her wheelchair and walker. Richelle described having to use a lot of trial and error and continued asking herself, "How can I make this easier and faster?" She shared that focusing on efficiency and the process of getting better and better was never burdensome for her, likely due to having Maximizer as one of her top strengths.

Look for things that can be improved
Pay attention to opportunities to improve processes, systems, or medical procedures during your cancer experience. Many advancements in cancer care stem from cancer survivors who have advocated for medical improvements, invented products, written books, or created nonprofits. You love the concept of good to great. What are you seeing that could be bumped up a notch? This could be anything from how the waiting room is set up to the packet of materials you receive as a new patient. You can express your feedback in online surveys or even more directly with your oncologist or a nurse navigator. You would make an excellent champion for a cancer cause, such as encouraging colonoscopy screenings, as well as a stellar advocate in the political arena. You know there is always room for growth, improvement, and getting better. Playing a part in improving processes, products, patient care, and outcomes will give you an instant boost and hopefully improve the cancer experience of many to follow.

I have benefited from the creativity of cancer survivor Diane Ungers LeBleu. After her bilateral mastectomy and experiencing discomfort with her surgical drains, Diane developed Pink Pockets™ to help people avoid using safety pins to attach their drains to hospital gowns, garments, and lanyards during showers.[56] Diane and her twin sister, Denise, have both survived breast cancer, and worked together on designing Pink Pockets™. As their website says, "Safety pins and pain pills do not mix. Pinning and unpinning these clumsy drains several times a day can be maddening for both patients and caregivers." Pink Pockets™ are worn inside your clothing and help you feel normal and comfortable for a fraction of the cost of other expensive drain solutions. A fellow survivor, Angie, gifted me Pink Pockets™ prior to my double mastectomy. I also used them for delayed breast reconstruction DIEP flap surgery. They are one of my go-to gifts for others undergoing major surgeries, and it's so cool that Diane took her pain and turned it into purpose with a product that has helped thousands of survivors.

Be Selective

People with the strength of Maximizer are naturally selective. They are typically pretty good at narrowing things down to the best. This can be anything from choosing the best breakfast spot on a beach vacation, the best photograph from a series, or the best group of people to support you during a medical crisis.

Laura is a Gallup-Certified Strengths Coach based in Dubai who endured a horrific life event when she was hit by a car while out for a run. She shared, "I can't emphasize enough how important it was for me to feel in control of my environment at times where everything felt overwhelming, painful, unknown and stressful. I need to feel that I am in the driving seat, focusing my efforts on what I can do best to positively impact my recovery. My Maximizer strength motivates me to keep going and reach those outcomes."

Laura recalls lying on the ground while panicked people huddled around her saying, "Stay with us." The accident caused her right foot to come off, her left foot to be completely smashed, a broken elbow, fractured wrist and ribs, and dislocated fingers. She used a wheelchair for five months and has so far undergone over 20 surgeries to regain her health

---

56 Pink Pockets™, Post Mastectomy Drain Holders: www.pink-pockets.com.

and mobility. Her journey to recovery continues. In her book, *Rebuilt to Last: Choose to Flourish*,[57] she shares that Maximizer is her top strength and she used that strength when relying on family and friends as caregivers and supporters. Laura shared, "Be selective. Surround yourself with people who help you succeed. I like to be with people who push me to be my best self. There is no doubt that I have overcome so much medical trauma because I have been so lucky to have excellent people around me. Whilst some of my closest friends are scattered across the globe, they have a big impact on how I feel and how I cope. They've sat by my bedside, held my hand, cheered me on and made me laugh. Together, they've helped me celebrate my wins. I feel blessed. My life is richer for them."

Delegate tasks that fit your supporters' strengths
If you have a solid support system like Laura, look for ways to involve them by delegating tasks that drain your energy. If you want to take it a step further, delegate tasks to just the right person to deliver based on their talents and strengths. For example, if you have a friend who loves socializing, invite them to drive you to one of your appointments and keep you company in the car and waiting room. If you have a friend with a child the same age as yours, ask them if they can help with a few car rides after school so you can take a power nap instead.

Cancer Cautions

Be gentle with yourself
Be careful not to hold yourself to too high of a standard as a cancer survivor. You will not be excellent every day. Although you use your Maximizer strength to push yourself to get better and better, now is not the time to be overly critical of yourself. Depending on the type of treatment you're receiving, you may have a variety of side effects from fatigue to nausea to body aches. Adjust your high expectations of yourself. You may

---

57 Everest, L. (2021) *Rebuilt to Last: Choose to Flourish*, Notion Press.

not be able to do the same things with the same level of quality as you were able to do prior to your diagnosis.

Share your high expectations with your care team
You have high expectations and may not be satisfied with the outcomes that many people feel are "just fine," or "good enough." Be prepared to honor your desire for the best outcomes and high-quality performance while you face cancer. Ask your care team members questions about how you can increase your odds of achieving the best outcomes. Be open to their insights around when to temper your expectations or adjust your definition of "best" when necessary for your recovery.

Positivity

People exceptionally talented in the Positivity theme have contagious enthusiasm. They are naturally upbeat and can energize others.

> I want my kids to know resilience is something we're about. We look on the sunny side of the street. We look for what's right, not what's wrong.
>
> —Hoda Kotb, American broadcast journalist and cancer survivor

You are generous with praise, quick to smile and have a naturally positive outlook. People want to be around you because your enthusiasm is contagious, and you make their world look better. Those who don't have your optimism sometimes find their world dull with repetition or heavy with pressure when bad things happen. You find a way to reassure them and lighten their spirit. You bring positive energy to every project, celebrate every achievement, and find ways to make everything more exciting. Some cynics may reject your optimism, but you are rarely dragged down. Your Positivity won't allow it. You believe that it is good to be alive, work can be fun, and no matter what the setbacks, everything will be OK.

Characteristics of Those with Positivity Talents

Fun	Hopeful	Giddy	Enthusiastic
Joyful	Dramatic	Optimistic	Positive-minded
Generous	Happy	Energetic	Influential
Lighthearted			

Cancer Connection

You are used to making an impression on people with your natural energy, enthusiasm, and inclination to make the most of life. As a cancer survivor, be prepared for this awe from others to be magnified. Your friends and loved ones have always been encouraged by your cheery disposition and great attitude. They may even have a hard time believing your diagnosis since they usually associate you with happiness and fun times. While you may have stretches of anger, worry, or sadness through your cancer experience, you will also probably bring hope and optimism along the way.

Ashley, a rectal cancer survivor diagnosed at 24, shared her viewpoint as a young cancer survivor with the Positivity strength. "When I was first diagnosed, and throughout treatment, of course, I shed many tears and had some down-in-the-dumps days. However, overall, I felt very positive about my journey and continue to feel that way today. During treatment, I would take it one day at a time or sometimes one hour at a time, but I knew treatment would eventually come to an end. Since then, I have remained positive about my future and health. I enjoy life and understand the gift that life is. When I was going through treatment, I remember being so frustrated when people would complain about *having to go to work or having to take their kids to practice*. When I hear these phrases today, I am quick to say, 'No, you GET to go to work. You GET to take the kids to practice.' There are so many people in this world that would love to have a normal work day or have the opportunity to have children but are not able to because of their devastating cancer diagnosis."

Positivity isn't high on my list of strengths. It's about middle of the pack, but I have had people assume that it's one of my top strengths, likely because I see the good in others and am fairly positive when it comes to human beings. So, it didn't surprise me too much when people recommended that I journal when I was diagnosed with cancer. As I mentioned in the introduction, there's a lot of advice out there for cancer survivors and it can be overwhelming. I felt like some advice was really helpful to me and other advice felt like it should be helpful. Take journaling, for example. I bet it is beneficial for some cancer survivors to jot down things they are grateful for, clear their thoughts, or capture ideas. But for whatever reason, as I was in the thick of my cancer treatment, that advice felt intimidating and stressful to me. I would have spent more time thinking, "What type of journal should I buy? What markers do real journalers use? Who is going to see this? What's the point?" So you can probably tell by the tone of my questions that I sometimes take things too seriously and focus more on the end game and the grade than the process. I remember, when I was sick, thinking that Positivity would be a pretty great strength to have while walking through cancer.

I had a theory that people with Positivity would be more likely to agree with, or even say, all those feisty phrases you hear and probably would enjoy journaling and focusing on gratitude. Josie, a breast cancer survivor validated my theory by sharing the following:

> Gratitude. It's almost overused nowadays but—dang! There is healing in looking around at all the people that love you. I have so much to be grateful for, and I make a list every single day. I'm grateful that I know how to help other people navigate hard diagnoses. I'm grateful that I know what really matters. I'm grateful for the new relationships that have formed. I'm grateful that my teens can look back and have memories of how strong our family was through hard times. Our family mantra for the last year was "stronger than before."

One cancer survivor I've often thought of when I considered the strength of Positivity is Hoda Kotb, the American broadcast journalist and former co-anchor of the NBC News morning show Today. She was diagnosed with Stage 1 breast cancer unexpectedly in her early forties and has 18 years of survivorship under her belt. I would bet my house on Hoda having Positivity as a top strength if she took the assessment. If you're a fan of the show or are one of her three million followers on Instagram, you would probably bet your house too. She just radiates fun, joy, and happiness. Her two adopted daughters are Haley Joy and Hope Catherine, names themselves that project Positivity.

As part of an *E! News* series called *What I Wish I Knew*,[58] Hoda shared, "I want my kids to know resilience is something we're about. We look on the sunny side of the street. We look for what's right, not what's wrong." When she discusses how cancer impacted her dream of carrying children of her own, she adds, "My best years of my life were all post cancer. God put them in my life at the perfect time. I will let them know about [my cancer] because we get stronger in the broken places. They were out there waiting for me, and I was waiting for them, and we came together just when we were supposed to." You can hear the optimism in her words, and her TV audiences felt the warmth and positive energy from her face over the decades. While she has been generous in sharing about her cancer experience every October during Breast Cancer Awareness Month, it is easy to forget about this challenging part of her life since she fills the TV screen with smiles, laughter, and fun energy. That may be part of her plan, as she has shared, "Cancer shaped me, but it did not define me. It's part of me, but not all of me."[59] She added, "But what you'll find is you're braver, you're more resilient."[60]

---

58 Mike Vulpo and Alex Ross, *E! News*. "Hoda Kotb—What I Wish I Knew Before My Battle with Breast Cancer." Available at: https://www.eonline.com/news/1352249/hoda-kotb-what-i-wish-i-knew-before-my-battle-with-breast-cancer.

59 A. Pawlowski, *Today* (October 4, 2024). "Hoda Kotb's Powerful Advice About Breast Cancer and 4 Words That Became Her Mantra. Available at: https://www.today.com/health/breast-cancer/hoda-kotb-breast-cancer-advice-rcna173844.

60 Vanessa Etienne and Lizzie Hyman, *People* (April 25, 2025). "Hoda Kotb Says Breast Cancer Is 'Part of Me, but Not All of Me.'" Available at: https://people.com/hoda-kotb-breast-cancer-changed-me-exclusive-11688545.

Positivity is a strength you can see, hear, and feel. No matter how you direct your Positivity, remind yourself that you have this warm energy and bright light within you. Use it to your advantage when your diagnosis, treatment, or survivorship days feel cold or dark. As my Strengths teacher, Curt Liesveld, shared:

> I help people appreciate a strength by saying, "What would happen if we could magically drain this from humanity?" And I think if we would drain Positivity from humanity, there would be less smiles. I've been to several places around the world. A smile is a universal language. In every culture, a smile means the same thing. That's one of the things that this theme brings to the world . . . joy, laughter, and smiling. We could all use a bit more of that.[61]

Cancer Considerations

Encourage your supporters to be optimistic
You can set the emotional tone for your cancer experience. If you want people to be optimistic, tell them so. Emphasize that, although this is going to be a challenge, you plan to focus on all the good things in life happening alongside your cancer diagnosis and treatment. You may need to request that your supporters do the same, as not everybody has your strength of Positivity.

Offer small acts of recognition
You are naturally talented at acknowledging and recognizing people, events, and experiences. Who would you like to recognize during your cancer experience? Are you seeing great things from your care team, your children, colleagues at work who step up, or your supporters? Don't put

---

61 Gallup CliftonStrengths. "Positivity: Learning to Love All 34 Talent Themes." Available at: https://www.gallup.com/cliftonstrengths/en/251261/positivity-learning-love-talent-themes.aspx.

pressure on yourself to do anything extraordinary. A handwritten note or an extra phone call would be a great form of recognition. They will be blown away that you are enduring cancer and taking time to recognize their actions. Jennifer is a breast cancer and brain tumor survivor who leans into her glass-half-full attitude to create moments of energy and encouragement. When she finished her last round of radiation, she gave her Duke University care team snack baskets to show her appreciation. Additionally, as she was about to be taken in for her brain biopsy, Jennifer lightened the seriousness in the room by asking the medical team, "Have you eaten and are you well hydrated? No 'hangry' people should be drilling into my head." She shared that the smiles created in that moment are forever burned into her memory. Jennifer's circle often tells her that she is the strongest person they know, and she believes this is due to her Positivity strength. She acknowledged that there are obviously times when she's not feeling strong and energetic, but she uses her Positivity strength to get refocused and return the optimism to every situation.

Help people know you are ready to face this
While Positivity is certainly about looking at things from the glass-half-full perspective, it is also about looking for solutions. You acknowledge your current reality and may have gotten to that point more quickly than your supporters. While some people may want to discuss what caused your disease, what treatment looked like in the past, or the shortcomings of the current healthcare system, you may not see much of a point. Your Positivity talent may help you move through that stage faster than others. You will be ready to look at the current state of your cancer diagnosis, understand the options on the table, and make the best decision for you and your family. Share your perspective and encourage others to join you in focusing on solutions and outcomes.

Plan to build some fun into the timeline
Your positive energy brings a boost to others around you. How can you incorporate fun and lighthearted activities into your life while going through your cancer experience? Is there a milestone you would like to

celebrate? Are you going to ring that bell when you finish chemotherapy or radiation treatments? Make the most of these exciting experiences you create. They will fill your bucket, and people will line up by your side to show their support.

Cancer Cautions

Beware of negativity
You can get dragged down by negative people. If there are people like that in your life, you may need to have an honest conversation to let them know what will help you most. That could also look like proactively sharing how you are approaching cancer with a positive outlook and mindset and invite them to join you. If you continue to sense negativity, this may be the time to set boundaries and possibly spend less time with them.

Communicate your optimism
People may think you are sugarcoating your cancer diagnosis due to your positive nature. Let them know that you understand the seriousness of the disease. Share that an overwhelming amount of negativity is not good for your mind, body, or spirit. Explain that you plan to take an optimistic approach to your health, treatment plan, and medical conversations and share some examples of what that looks like for you.

Relator

People exceptionally talented in the Relator theme enjoy close relationships. They find deep satisfaction in working hard with friends to achieve a goal.

Relator describes how you develop and maintain relationships. As a Relator, you gravitate toward people you already know and trust. You do not necessarily shy away from meeting new people, but you do derive a great deal of pleasure and strength from being around your closest friends. For you, a relationship has value only if it is genuine. Once you make a meaningful connection with someone, you actively nurture the relationship to make it stronger and deeper. You want to understand the other person's feelings, their goals, their fears, and their dreams, and you want them to understand yours. You know that this kind of closeness might make you vulnerable and put you at risk, but you are willing to take that risk. The more you share with each other, the more you risk together. The more you risk together, the more each of you proves you genuinely care.

> I took my husband and the same four friends with me to every chemotherapy appointment.
>
> —Angie, breast cancer survivor

Characteristics of Those with Relator Talents

Friendly	Authentic	Intimate
Truthful	Caring	Genuine
Transparent	Revealing	

Cancer Connection

With your Relator strength, you likely prefer to keep things authentic, genuine, and casual. *Keep it real* may be a quote that resonates with you. Although Relator is one of the most frequently occurring of the 34 strengths, some people won't have this strength and may be less comfortable having conversations with you about your cancer diagnosis. Recognize that and encourage people to continue to treat you the way they did as your friend, colleague, or family member. You may want them to acknowledge your cancer diagnosis and fold that right into what they already knew about you rather than tiptoeing around the topic or treating you like you're a completely different person given this one change in your life.

If your cancer diagnosis slows you down, potentially impacting the number of hours you're available for work or other commitments, find other ways to build time connecting with people into your schedule. You may prefer face-to-face time with people but defer to phone calls or video conferencing if you must, as some connection is better than none for you.

You value genuineness and authenticity. The healthcare arena may feel a bit cold and sterile to you. Remind yourself that even though you typically aren't interested in building relationships with people you may never see or talk to again, the people you encounter in the waiting rooms are part of the vast humanness that makes life fascinating. This could help you tolerate the otherwise bland, boring settings and routine appointments.

Waiting rooms can also be places for connecting. I had some of my best conversations with my close girlfriends in the infusion center waiting room. We shared laughs and tears discussing topics ranging from our kids to our parents to some love and loss we'd each experienced over the years. The conversations were not about my cancer diagnosis, but they were real and deep and so beautiful. Find the beauty in the people and places you connect more deeply with through this health experience.

Cancer Considerations

Seek a trusted confidant

You are great at building long and deep relationships. You may still be friends with people you grew up with such as neighborhood and high school friends. Your cancer diagnosis will introduce new people into your life, like it or not. You will likely have a multifaceted care team surrounding you, and you may be introduced to other cancer survivors along the way. Pay close attention to these new relationships. Is there a care team member or cancer survivor you'd like to build a relationship with beyond simple professionalism? You may flourish by having one or two trusted confidants who can speak this new language of cancer fluently with you. This will help your cancer experience feel less lonely and abstract and more real and vulnerable, just the way you approach life and relationships.

Build trust with your care team

You may enjoy being part of a team and working toward a shared goal. Picture your medical providers in the same uniform or jersey as you and playing on the same team. Instead of thinking of them as superior, or as outside advisers, think of them as colleagues, peers, and team members. That mindset shift will help you build trust with them sooner.

Chris, a Stage 3 melanoma cancer survivor, used his Relator strength to build relationships with his care team while gaining a deep understanding about his health challenges. Chris shared, "My medical team had half-hour appointments with me, and they'd spend an hour with me instead. I had an opportunity to go to another excellent center for treatment, but I'm not sure I'd have had the same relationships at that larger center."

Inner circle of support

You may have circles or clusters of friends with common histories or interests. On Gallup's *Theme Thursday* podcast, Curt Liesveld, who has Relator in his Top 5, shared, "There's almost a freedom that you have when you're with those people who know you best and love you most. I feel more at home."[62] Are there certain circles you want to invite into your cancer experience to feel more at home? Or are there specific people in those circles you want to spend more time with? Angie, a breast cancer survivor, smiled as she reflected on her treatment experience. "I took the same four friends with me to every chemotherapy appointment." With the strength of Relator, Angie knew that she wanted to keep her inner circle close to her during those challenging times as a young mother diagnosed with cancer in her thirties.

Invite your friends in for the tough stuff

You may be a casual or more informal person who doesn't put on a shiny exterior or pretend to be someone you're not. You are often the one other people go to with their problems, so they may not be used to the role reversal. Your close circles of friends may be struggling with your cancer diagnosis, what to say, what to ask, and how to help. Your relaxed style may help put them at ease and reassure your supporters that you are still you, despite this new diagnosis and health challenge ahead. Feel free to ask open-ended questions like "How are you feeling about all of this?" or "What questions do you have about my diagnosis?" You are opening the door and inviting them into a more personal, real experience together with you in working through your cancer experience.

Consider who needs to know

You may prefer to keep your experience semiprivate by sharing only with your selected inner circle of friends and family. One cancer survivor, Deb,

---

62 Gallup CliftonStrengths. "Relator: Learning to Love All 34 Talent Themes." Available at: https://www.gallup.com/cliftonstrengths/en/251381/relator-learning-love-talent-themes.aspx.

has the strength of Relator and shared that she created a CaringBridge web page for her close circle. Deb added, "This helped me connect and stay connected with those who are important to me." Another survivor with the Relator strength added, "I kept my circle of people who knew about my diagnosis very small."

Cancer Cautions

Appointments may feel too brief
Unfortunately, there may be medical appointments where time is limited, or your provider is running behind schedule. Given your desire to build deep relationships with people, be prepared to leave a few appointments wanting more time together. To make the most of the time you do have, prepare opening questions and more detailed questions in advance. Write these down in a notebook or in your phone and skip the small talk about the weather during these early meetings. To build deeper relationships with your providers, you can always follow up with additional questions or a thank-you in the online medical portal if that feels helpful to you.

Give people time to catch up
Some people are not as comfortable with deep, intimate conversations as you. You have probably noticed that over the years, but their unease may be magnified when it comes to your cancer diagnosis and health updates. Do your best to draw them in if you want them to get more vulnerable about how they're feeling but be prepared for these conversations to take longer, initially, to allow others to get comfortable with the increased intimacy.

Responsibility

People exceptionally talented in the Responsibility theme take psychological ownership of their commitments. They are dependable and embrace values such as honesty and loyalty.

> If the oncologist made a recommendation, I listened. I was a dutiful, conscientious patient.
>
> —Melissa, breast cancer survivor

You take psychological ownership for anything you commit to, and whether large or small, you feel emotionally bound to follow it through to completion. Your good name depends on it. If for some reason you cannot deliver, apologies are not enough. Excuses and rationalizations are unacceptable. You will not quite be able to live with yourself until you have made restitution. Your conscientiousness, your obsession for doing things right, and your impeccable ethics combine to create your reputation: utterly dependable. When people come to you for help—and they will—you must be selective. Your willingness to volunteer may sometimes cause you to take on more than you should.

Characteristics of Those with Responsibility Talents

Diligent	Judgmental	Driven	Dependable
Committed	Responsive	Conscientious	Loyal
Dutiful	Serious	Self-sacrificing	Independent

Cancer Connection

People with Responsibility as a strength are loyal, dependable, and reliable. You often get things done because you told somebody that you would. You are a person of your word. You are motivated to follow through because feeling valued and committed is energizing to you. As you move through your cancer experience, you will need to examine your responsibilities, priorities, and the new demands on your time. People with the Responsibility strength typically keep full schedules and have lots of commitments. You probably already had plenty on your plate to accomplish, and adding a cancer diagnosis to the equation requires you to adjust. Honor the reality that although your diagnosis probably requires an adjustment, it may not mean you have to stop everything. Sometimes keeping things on your plate is a form of coping, feeling purposeful, and directing energy toward the positive. One cancer survivor shared, "I know when I didn't feel good, I honored my body's need to heal and didn't work, or worked a reduced day. But I also had enough self-awareness to understand that my psyche needed me to work whenever I felt up to it, and that felt really good."

You may notice a shift in your focus from external to internal as you navigate cancer. While you are typically responding to the requests of others, now is a critical time to turn toward your own needs. Meeting with physicians, learning new terminology, reviewing medical results, and making decisions takes a lot of time and energy. These new demands need your full attention and focus.

Recognize your unique ability to honor commitments and take your duties seriously, like following your medication regimen, tracking vitals, or eating a prescribed diet. One melanoma cancer survivor shared, "If the doctor told me to change my diet, I changed my diet. If I was to lift my arm 10 times, I lifted my arm. If I was told to rest, I made sure to rest. They knew I would do what was asked of me." Dr. Melissa Reade, a breast cancer survivor, shared that she has followed all the rules and completed her homework. "If the oncologist made a recommendation, I listened. I was a dutiful, conscientious patient. If you have this Responsibility strength, I'd recommend that you ask questions, get clear on what's expected of you, and follow through on those asks."

Find ways to celebrate and appreciate your diligence and persistence, such as treating yourself with a small reward like a new book or pair of walking shoes. You will be an ideal, compliant, vigilant patient, and your health will benefit as you keep your incredible track record of following through on commitments. If they were handing out grades to cancer survivors, you get an A+ for your follow-through.

Cancer Considerations

What can you let go?
Conduct a careful analysis of where you spend your time. Review your to-do lists and calendar over the last few months. You may have your hands in many pots, from work to home to organizations to your community. Your health trumps most of your commitments. You prepare the monthly meeting minutes as secretary for a nonprofit board? No problem. The board either survives a few months without them or somebody else can capture the minutes. You organize coffee and donuts for your faith community? Also, no problem. Pass the torch to another member. In fact, many commitments can be delayed, modified, or handled by somebody else. Since you are used to delivering on promises, reducing your commitments and letting things go may be hard and humbling, even though you know it will be in the best interest of your health.

What responsibilities serve you?

What responsibilities do you still WANT to own and complete? Now is the time to be selective about your commitments. You enjoy freedom and autonomy in completing your work, so try to create that where possible. Melissa shared it was important for her to continue driving her young children to school each day. People offered to do this for her, but this was not an activity where she wanted support. It was important for her to continue this parenting routine, for her personal fulfillment and for her children to retain some sense of normalcy and life before Mom had cancer.

Get creative to make it work

If it's important to you to continue traveling for your job or volunteering at the local pet shelter, what steps do you need to take for that to be possible, given your treatment plan? Maybe it means you need to go to sleep one hour earlier each night or take it easy on the weekends. Your bucket is filled by following through on your commitments, so you should continue to act and serve where you're able if it gives you a boost of energy and purpose. But you must be clear about which obligations are most important to you and what adjustments you need to make so you don't exhaust yourself when you need to rest and heal.

Delegate

If you're not already an expert at delegating, now is the time to up your game. Develop a habit of evaluating your schedule and workload consistently looking for things that can be handled by somebody else. If you're working and able to continue during treatment, schedule time with your supervisor to brainstorm ways to reduce your workload. Depending on your industry and role, this may give your direct report, a mentee, or another colleague a great developmental opportunity to step up and provide support. If you have children, consider shifting some of your responsibilities to your partner, spouse, or another child where age appropriate. This could be the perfect time for other family members to mow the lawn, vacuum the cars, grocery shop, water the plants, or cook a meal.

Research available support

If you need assistance with meals or cleaning, there may be nonprofits in your community that provide this type of support. In Iowa, Can Do Cancer[63] is an amazing nonprofit organization that works to enhance the lives of breast cancer patients through providing dinner on chemotherapy days, monthly house cleaning services while in treatment, and a website of resources. Ask your medical care team for a list of organizations or resources that provide similar support. While you are typically used to doing a lot of work and getting things done on your own, now is the time to delegate and ask for help from your supporters.

One cancer survivor shared with me, "I enlisted the help of friends to take my kids to do something fun, like go to a park or play mini putt. I also had my husband's friends take him out for breaks from all things cancer." If you are a caretaker to a family member, evaluate if you'll have the ability or energy to continue the same level of care. Secure help to take care of your loved one from other family members, close friends, a medical facility, or in-home nursing care if necessary.

Make your health and energy a top priority

Work to understand the behaviors, activities, and practices that will improve your physical and mental health. Establish your health-related priorities and create some nonnegotiables, if necessary. Your morning walk or alone time for meditation may be nonnegotiables on your daily agenda. Pay close attention to what activities and people are receiving your energy. How do you feel during these experiences? If they are depleting your energy, or you anticipate they will, you may need to create a boundary. Some people report they gained clarity around their friendships and where they wanted to spend their precious time after experiencing cancer. You are used to others describing you as reliable and dependable. Make sure you are also making yourself a priority and delivering on promises you've made to yourself.

---

63 Can Do Cancer: https://candocancer.org.

Consider (but don't yet commit to) chances to give back
There are so many opportunities to get involved and give back to the cancer community. Take note of any organizations or opportunities that strike your interest. Your ability to follow through on commitments will make you a great cancer mentor, event volunteer, policy advocate, or other service-related role. If you are asked to participate in a cancer-related outlet, take your time to consider the opportunity before saying *yes*. Don't rush into these decisions as they are rarely urgent. You may have the heart for volunteering or advocacy, but make sure you also have the energy and time before you commit.

Cancer Cautions

Don't blame yourself
You did not ask for cancer. This isn't something you agreed to incorporate into your already full life. It is an unfortunate health challenge. Work to remove, or at least reduce, the amount of guilt you may feel related to your diagnosis. For most cancers, it is difficult to pinpoint the exact cause of the disease. Depending on your type of cancer, potential contributing factors may range from genetics to environmental contaminants to lifestyle choices to unknown factors.

People with the strength of Responsibility take serious ownership of their actions. Be careful how much ownership you take of the *why* behind your diagnosis, especially if there isn't a direct correlation or cause-and-effect relationship to your type of cancer. As a breast cancer survivor, I could beat myself up for a variety of things from the foods I ate to having children later in life at 30 and 36. My cancer was not genetic, and my care team couldn't pinpoint the cause. Mentally torturing myself over behaviors that may or may not have contributed to this disease would have been a poor coping mechanism.

Many cancer survivors must deal with ambiguity about the cause of their cancer. If you need help working through guilt or shame, seek guidance from a counselor, therapist, support group, or fellow cancer survivor. It may be helpful to pursue multiple avenues of support to process these strong emotions.

Avoid obsessing over decision-making
Keep in mind that there is not a singular right way to approach cancer. You tend to be a serious person who values integrity and reliability. While this is an advantage for you as you carefully evaluate your options and work to make the right decision, be careful not to obsess over making the wrong one. You'll make hundreds of decisions and yours may differ from those of other cancer survivors you meet or learn about, and that's okay. In fact, there are so many variables involved in cancer survivorship that you may never know exactly which decisions impacted your health outcomes.

Focus on what you can do
Failing to deliver on commitments is not an option in your mind. Try not to hold yourself to unrealistic expectations of what you can accomplish with cancer as a new part of your life. Work to focus on the quality of what you can do, instead of on the quantity of how much you used to do. You are motivated by people viewing you as dependable, so be careful not to keep or add too many commitments to the detriment of your healing.

Restorative

People exceptionally talented in the Restorative theme are adept at dealing with problems. They are good at figuring out what is wrong and resolving it.

You love to solve problems. Some people are discouraged by setbacks and breakdowns, but you are energized by them. You enjoy the challenge of analyzing the symptoms, identifying what is wrong, and finding the solution. You may prefer practical problems or conceptual ones or personal ones. You may seek out specific kinds of problems that you have seen before and that you are confident you can fix. Or you may feel the greatest thrill when faced with complex, unfamiliar problems. It is a wonderful feeling for you to restore something to its true glory, to bring it back to life. Intuitively, you know that without your intervention, this thing—this machine, this technique, this company—might have ceased to function. You fixed it, resuscitated it, rekindled its vitality. You saved it.

To some extent, getting to the final diagnosis was a relief for me. As someone who thrives at identifying and solving problems, the final diagnosis helped me laser focus on a path forward and formulate the plan with my doctors and the plan for my family.

—Kathy, lymphoma survivor

Characteristics of Those with Restorative Talents

Problem-oriented Investigative Responsive
Insightful Driven Weakness-oriented
Unintimidated

Cancer Connection

You may be somebody known to be a fixer; whether that's repairing broken things around the house, troubleshooting computer issues, or helping people with their problems. You see problems as part of life, and you may even view your cancer diagnosis the same way. While you may never have anticipated your diagnosis, you won't hesitate to jump in and address it. Keep in mind that most types of cancer take time to resolve or be "fixed," if possible. You may be used to quick fixes, so prepare yourself that it may take multiple steps to thoroughly diagnosis this problem, let alone solve it. Unfortunately, some forms of cancer diagnoses are terminal and may not be able to be reversed, but there are still ways for those survivors to take an investigative and determined approach to their care.

Kathy was diagnosed with lymphoma and has Restorative as her top strength. She investigated multiple paths while waiting to receive an official diagnosis and shared this:

> We knew something was wrong. I had a lump and nerve pain, an inconclusive biopsy, and then a surgery. But we still didn't know what specific problem we were faced with yet. My sister and I had done a lot of research, reaching out to people we knew in the oncology and autoimmune fields and taking the data we could gather from test results and using it to plan for various scenarios. To some extent, getting to the final diagnosis was a relief for me. As someone who thrives at identifying and solving problems, the final diagnosis helped me laser focus on a path forward and formulate the plan with my doctors and the plan for my family.

> You go through a lot of emotions getting to a diagnosis. You hope it isn't cancer and then get used to cancer being on the table. Then you hope it isn't certain kinds of cancer or that it hasn't spread too far and then get used to those being possibilities. It is emotionally, physically, and mentally draining. Our research and consideration of multiple paths helped me be in a better mental state when the diagnosis came through. I accepted it and faced it head on. Having the information in advance allowed me to research and plan, prepare questions, and be fully present when meeting with my oncologist for the first time. It changed the conversation from me trying to absorb what was going on to me being in action mode.

Restorative falls in the Executing domain, and you can hear a lot of hard work, intensity, and resiliency coming through in Kathy's words. If you recall my own story, from the introduction to this book, you may remember me mentioning that I taught a class at ACT the morning of my cancer diagnosis. Kathy was my awesome client counterpart and walked me to my workshop that morning on the ACT campus and many more workshops to follow. In the months ahead, my appearance changed as chemo took my hair, weakened my immunity, and slashed my energy levels. I'll always remember how incredibly supportive Kathy was during this tough stretch, no doubt in part due to her strength in managing difficulties and pushing forward successfully.

Cancer Considerations

Spread the calm
You may be calmer than others when dealing with treatment delays, medical setbacks, or difficult side effects. Your innate knowledge that problems are part of the deal will serve you well as you spend hours in waiting rooms, exam rooms, infusion chairs, or radiation centers. If you think it is appropriate, share your mindset with others waiting around you. Your

practical mindset may be just the influence they need to shift their energy from annoyed and disappointed to calm and accepting.

What needs fixing?

You may want to help other people with cancer. As you learn more about cancer-related organizations or public policy, pay attention to what things stand out to you as something that needs fixing. For example, you may learn that some cancer survivors are unable to find rides to treatment and that some organizations, like the American Cancer Society Road to Recovery® program, provide this service.[64] This may tug on your heartstrings, so you decide to volunteer to be a driver once your health has improved. Or you may learn about specific policies that would help cancer survivors save time and reduce healthcare costs, such as Biomarker Testing. According to the American Cancer Society, "Biomarker testing is an important step for accessing precision medicine including targeted therapies that can lead to improved survivorship and better quality of life for cancer patients."[65] You might find that fascinating and decide to get involved with advocacy work to help solve tangible problems impacting thousands of people.

Focus on what is in your control

Depending on the type of cancer you have, you may not know what caused the disease. As badly as you will want to pinpoint that root cause, it may never be uncovered through genetic testing or determined by your care team. This ambiguity may frustrate you, but focus on what risk factors you can troubleshoot. For example, age, diet, and exercise levels may be risk factors involved with your type of cancer. While you can't control growing older and aging, you can impact the food you eat and the number of minutes you exercise weekly. You may question if environmental

---

64 American Cancer Society, American Cancer Society Road to Recovery® program. Available at: https://www.cancer.org/support-programs-and-services/road-to-recovery.html.

65 American Cancer Society Cancer Action Network. Available at: https://www.fightcancer.org/what-we-do/access-biomarker-testing.

factors influenced your diagnosis such as the air or water quality near your home. Even without a clear cause-and-effect relationship you can point to for your cancer, remind yourself that taking steps to improve your health is always a step in the right direction.

Cancer Cautions

Monitor your mindset
Be aware of how focusing on the problems related to your diagnosis or treatment impacts your energy levels, mindset, and well-being. If it leads you toward negativity, regroup and reframe how you see and process your cancer-related issues or setbacks in a more positive way. You may want to enlist a member of your care team or a therapist to talk through what you're feeling to get their perspective. They may be able to share statistics or examples to help you understand if your cancer-related challenges are rare, common, will improve on their own, or need to be proactively solved.

Avoid rushing to fix things
You may be putting energy and emotion toward fixing a problem that is a common side effect and will resolve on its own. For example, chemotherapy may impact your appetite and lead you to want smoothies over solid foods. As a natural problem solver, your gut instinct may be to purchase an expensive smoothie maker. However, your oncologist or another cancer survivor may share with you that the appetite change will be short-lived and your desire to eat solid food will return soon. By gaining more insight and information, you may save yourself time and energy from researching smoothie makers, as well as money and counter space.

Don't criticize yourself
You are good at seeing things that need to be fixed. Don't lump yourself into a weak or broken category just because you aren't running with a full tank of gas. No matter how smoothly your treatment goes, you may still

experience fatigue, sickness, or emotional distress. Don't be too critical of yourself for experiencing expected side effects. Consider exploring mindfulness practices through the work of Zen Master Thich Nhat Hanh,[66] self-compassion exercises from Dr. Kristin Neff,[67] or other meditations or calming practices. Thich Nhat Hanh is a global spiritual leader, the "Father of Mindfulness," who wrote over 100 books on mindfulness and has millions of followers across the world. Dr. Neff's work teaches us that "Self-compassion simply involves doing a U-Turn and giving yourself the same compassion you'd naturally show a friend. It means being supportive when you're facing a life challenge." The most important thing for you to do is rest and recover.

Be patient

You may not ever feel fully fixed or repaired after your cancer diagnosis. Even with the best possible treatment outcomes, many cancer survivors say their lives are never the same after their diagnosis. They may have lingering side effects from chemotherapy, radiation, surgery, or medication. Additionally, the mental challenges of navigating cancer survivorship may impact you for months and years. Be patient with your progress and consider that restoring yourself to Life Before Cancer may not be as realistic as becoming the 2.0 version of yourself. Jen, a mucosal melanoma cancer survivor with Restorative shared that "Recently, I've been focusing on this ongoing time, the gift of survivorship and not wasting that. Particularly for those of us whose cancers include close monitoring and regular scans forever, there is a feeling of never getting to a place of being fixed. It helps me to think that through cancer survivorship, we have been given something to make us stronger, if we take advantage of it."

---

66 Thich Nhat Hanh, Plum Village: https://plumvillage.org/about/thich-nhat-hanh.
67 Kristin Neff, Self-Compassion: https://self-compassion.org.

Self-Assurance

People exceptionally talented in the Self-Assurance theme feel confident in their ability to manage their own lives. They have an inner compass that gives them certainty in their decisions.

Self-Assurance is similar to self-confidence. You have faith in your strengths, and you own your decisions. You know that you are able to take risks, to meet new challenges, to stake claims, and, most important, to deliver. You push your own limits and look for challenges, confident you will conquer them. But Self-Assurance is more than self-confidence. Not only are you sure about your strengths and abilities, you also trust your judgment. When you look at the world, you know that your perspective is unique. You know that no one can make decisions for you because no one sees exactly what you see. No one can tell you what to think. They can guide. They can suggest. But you alone have the conviction to make decisions and act. Unlike some, you are not easily swayed by others' arguments, no matter how persuasive they may be.

The long-term side effects of treatment still creep into my life today. Even with those side effects, I have this confidence about me and know I can do hard things. I know I have been given a second chance at life, so I am not going to waste it.

—Ashley, rectal cancer survivor

Characteristics of Those with Self-Assurance Talents

Independent	Confident	Self-sufficient	Intense
Stable	Certain	Self-aware	Instinctive
Controlling	Persistent		

Cancer Connection

Self-Assurance is one of the rarest strengths in the world, according to Gallup data. While your cancer diagnosis may cause you to feel rattled, afraid, overwhelmed, and many other emotions, your strength is going to help you navigate this challenge better than many. Cancer survivors, regardless of the kind of cancer, are faced with one thing in common—the need to make a lot of decisions. The good news for you with your Self-Assurance strength is that you tend to be confident in your decisions. While you may be open to input or advice from others, whether it's your oncologist or life partner, you feel comfortable that the final call is up to you. People will be surprised with how well you move through the phases of receiving your diagnosis, undergoing treatment and focusing on your health and well-being. The reason for their surprise may very well be the fact that you have a talent that is rarely seen and makes you unique. Embrace this uniqueness of yours and remind yourself of this strength as you face many decisions during your cancer experience.

You like feeling in control of your life and making your own decisions. Cancer can certainly make you feel less in control. Upon receiving your diagnosis, remind yourself to control the controllables. While you can't control your illness, you can control the amount of information you consume about it. And you can control if you'd like to get a second or even third opinion from another cancer professional. And you can control who you tell about your diagnosis, when you tell them, and how you deliver the message. So, although your feeling of being in control may have been threatened by this diagnosis, remind yourself there are still many aspects of your health and well-being that are completely in your control. You will do very well operating under that mindset.

People with the Self-Assurance strength are self-aware and confident. Ashley was diagnosed with Stage 3 rectal cancer at the age of 24. Her treatment lasted one year and included 28 days of continuous IV chemotherapy with radiation daily, tumor resection with temporary ileostomy placement, and 12 cycles of additional chemotherapy. An ileostomy is an operation where the ileum portion of your small intestine is diverted to a surgically created opening in the abdomen wall "to provide a new path for waste material to leave the body."[68] Ashley shared, "When you go through a cancer diagnosis and treatment, the lucky ones can look back at the experience and say, 'Wow, I did it!' The long-term side effects of treatment still creep into my life today, such as pelvic floor dysfunction, neuropathy, and challenges with infertility." She continued, "However, even with those side effects, I have this confidence about me and know I can do hard things. I know I have been given a second chance at life, so I am not going to waste it." Since her diagnosis, Ashley was able to deliver two healthy boys with the help of in vitro fertilization. Her friends and family were impressed by her inner strength and confidence as she navigated her unexpected cancer diagnosis at such an early age. That admiration continues today, 13 years later, as they watch her prioritize her health through a nutritious diet and commitment to exercise and strength training.

Cancer Considerations

You'll feel confident in your own decisions
You are an excellent decision-maker and may select your course of action more quickly than many cancer survivors. Once you have the necessary information about your options, you will probably be ready to decide.

---

68   Ileostomy—NCI Dictionary of Cancer Terms: https://www.cancer.gov/publications/dictionaries/cancer-terms/def/ileostomy.

While "trusting your gut" is a big part of the strength of Self-Assurance,[69] you may still take steps to research, read books, or seek counsel. These steps will help you know you're making a wise decision. Other people may be more likely to count on guidance from others in reaching their final decision. You may consult with others but are less likely to rely on them for final decisions. Moving forward independently has usually worked out just fine for you. In fact, one guest on Gallup's *Theme Thursday* podcast shared, "I make decisions, and I'm prepared to live with them. Self-Assurance is about an inner capacity to know myself, trust myself, and trust my decisions and my approaches."

Reassure people

People close to you may be more scared, emotional, and overwhelmed than you. Reassure them that you have the information you need to make reasoned decisions. Explain that you have processed this diagnosis and understand its serious nature. Your calm and confident style will help build your supporters' trust in your plan and process too.

What can you delegate?

You are probably very self-aware and comfortable with who you are, what you know, and what is out of your wheelhouse. Are there aspects of your cancer diagnosis that you'd rather delegate out? You can't delegate your radiation, but maybe you need to find a store that sells wigs or a local physical therapist. If the thought of researching these options drains you, delegate that to somebody who wants to help. They may give you three final choices and your decision will be easy. You will spend a few minutes on that process start to finish instead of an hour or two of research and phone calls to get to the same outcome.

---

69 Gallup CliftonStrengths. "Self-Assurance: Learning to Love All 34 Talent Themes." Available at: https://www.gallup.com/cliftonstrengths/en/251405/self-assurance-learning-love-talent-themes.aspx.

Cancer Cautions

Remind yourself of past success
Don't lose faith in your gut and the mind–body connection you've likely felt most of your life. Some cancer survivors report feeling "betrayed by their body." Now is the time to get realigned with your gut instincts if you are feeling off-balance. Regroup and remind yourself of all the times in your life when your natural abilities and inner knowing have helped you make hard decisions and succeed.

Lean on others
You don't have to go this alone. Although you are used to being independent and in control, you don't have to remain that way through your cancer experience. You're surrounded by care team members and hopefully a solid support system. Lean on others when you need information, insights, advice, or help.

Significance

People exceptionally talented in the Significance theme want to make a big impact. They are independent and prioritize what will increase their influence on others or their organization.

I really feel like I'm a walking miracle. This experience left me with a voice saying, "There's a reason I'm still here. How can I make the most of it? How can I leave a legacy? How can I make a difference in the world?"

—Gina, neuroendocrine tumor survivor

You want other people to see you as significant. You want to be heard, to stand out, to be known and appreciated—especially for your unique strengths. You need others to admire you as credible, professional, and successful. Likewise, you want to associate with others who are credible, professional, and successful. If they aren't, you will push them until they are—or you will move on. As an independent spirit, you want your work to be a way of life rather than a job, and you want the freedom to do things your way. Your yearnings are intense, and your life is filled with goals, achievements, or qualifications you crave. Whatever your focus, your Significance theme will keep pulling you upward, away from the mediocre toward the exceptional. It is the theme that keeps you reaching.

Characteristics of Those with Significance Talents

Admired	Successful	Influential	Independent
Professional	Credible	Visible	Desirous
Exceptional	Audience-oriented		

Cancer Connection

People with the strength of Significance take life seriously and are motivated by meaningful ambitions and goals. Given your determination to make a difference, you tend to spend your time on things you feel are important. Many people gain clarity through cancer on what is a waste of time to do, and what really matters in their life. You probably already have that clarity. You are driven to make an impact, whether in your career, relationships, or community. This cancer diagnosis may even sharpen your focus on the contributions you want to make during your lifetime.

Significance is currently one of the rarest of the 34 CliftonStrengths so you may feel unique in your urge to excel and be viewed as successful, even as a cancer patient. You are likely somebody with a long list of goals and a drive to make a difference in the world. As a driven goal-getter with high expectations, some things may need to shift. Continue to maintain your focus on making a difference while also accepting that your goals, timelines, and workload may need adjusted. While your energy levels will likely be down, your desire to contribute and push toward your purpose will remain.

Dr. Giulia Bonaminio, a breast cancer survivor and the current Senior Associate Dean for Medical Education at the University of Kansas School of Medicine, shared with me that she had her surgery and radiation treatments within the medical community where she taught. She smiled big while sharing, "I was so happy to have them, now physicians, treat me. I'm really proud to have my former students as my care team." Dr. Bonaminio's passion for medical education and pride in the success of her students is a powerful example of her Significance strength. In an unexpected full circle moment, she was able to experience the tremendous care that the physicians who were her students provided. This experience was a nod to the impact she made on them and the ripple effect on the lives of all their patients.

Cancer Considerations

Seek out the best
You enjoy being in the company of accomplished and successful people. As you consider your cancer institution, oncologist, and care team options, which places and people meet your need to be healed by the best? Once you have selected a healthcare provider, ask questions about their education, certifications, and publications to assure you of their experience. Success fuels you, so let yourself go after the best care to inspire your healing.

Learn about patients with successful outcomes
Feedback from important people in your life motivates you to reach your goals. You genuinely care what they think about you and your performance. Ask your care team what you can do to excel at your treatment. What did their most successful patients with the same diagnosis do that might have led to their improved outcomes? These suggestions may range from diet and exercise shifts to managing sleep and stress. Consider all your options through the lens of making a significant contribution to your own healing. As your care progresses, gather feedback from your team on how your cancer is performing relative to other patients who experienced tremendous results. Ask if there is any action you can take to improve your health outcomes, and make the necessary adjustments based on their feedback. Not everything is in our control as cancer patients, but you'll naturally be curious about what you can do to move the needle in a positive direction.

Think about your legacy

Leaving a legacy is central to your identity. You are probably driven by a desire to not only succeed but to succeed at something you feel is important. Dr. Maya Angelou, poet, author, and civil rights activist, said, "If you're going to live, leave a legacy. Make a mark on the world that can't be erased."[70] Oprah Winfrey often shares that Dr. Maya Angelou told her, "You have no idea what your legacy will be because your legacy is every life you've touched."[71] I spoke with Gina, a Gallup-Certified Strengths Coach and cancer survivor with the strength of Significance. She shared how her health scare led to big reflections about her life and legacy.

> I had an experience where a great deal of pain led me to go to the emergency room. The GI doctor said I had diverticulitis and while in the waiting room, I asked the nurse to see the report. Although the nurse seemed annoyed and my husband gave me a little bit of a hard time, I felt like I needed to advocate for myself. When I looked at the report, it mentioned a tumor on my pancreas. I questioned the doctor, and he said it was probably nothing and to keep an eye on it for a few years. I went to a surgeon next, and he said the same thing. But when my husband asked what he would do if it was his wife, the surgeon replied that he'd probably take it out. So, I moved forward with surgery, and he removed one-third of my pancreas and my one-day hospital stay shifted to one week. The surgeon was floored by the size of the tumor and discovered it was cancerous. He said, "You guys knew something was off. You saved your life."
>
> I really feel like I'm a walking miracle and have a drive to tell my story. This experience left me with a voice saying, "There's a reason I'm still here. How can I make the most of it? How can I leave a legacy? How can I make a difference in the world?" I

---

70 Maya Angelou, Caged Bird Legacy: https://www.mayaangelou.com.
71 Oprah Winfrey, "What Oprah Knows for Sure About Being a Supportive Friend." https://www.oprah.com/inspiration/what-oprah-knows-for-sure-about-being-a-supportive-friend.

want to encourage others to advocate for themselves. Don't let your well-being sit in somebody else's hands.

If legacy resonates with you, consider if your cancer diagnosis impacts the difference you want to make in the world. As a natural difference-maker, do you have clarity on the big things you want to accomplish? Do you have a plan for the steps along the way? Reach out to your contacts if you'd appreciate help brainstorming ideas, narrowing your focus, or enlisting supporters to help you with your mission. People will line up to work with you on your priorities. If you prefer a neutral source, consider enlisting a psychologist, counselor, or coach to help you chart your path.

Hold onto your vision
Dr. Bonaminio explained that she was still very focused on her career during her cancer experience. She shared, "I've got work to do. I have a purpose. What I do is really important to me, and I enjoy it." It's important to hold onto your vision and drive even when you may need to take a rest. While your cancer diagnosis may disrupt your original pace, it doesn't have to derail your determination. Your ambition is an important part of you!

Focus of attention
You may be someone who naturally enjoys the spotlight, the microphone, and the stage. Prepare yourself to be a focal point of worried family, friends, and supporters as you navigate your diagnosis and treatment plan. While you typically may not shy away from playing the main character on center stage, now you can also serve as the lighting director and control what others see and hear about your health. Turn on the floodlights by sharing your medical updates, how you are feeling physically and emotionally, and asking for help from your many supporters. You may enjoy sharing cancer-related pictures and videos on social media, writing on your CaringBridge or other private website, or calling or texting friends to share updates.

Dim the lights when you don't want to be seen or your energy or emotions demand that you rest. You can delegate the communication tasks to a trusted friend or family member when necessary and read messages later when you need a boost. Don't allow your position in the spotlight at center stage to drain you; use it only to energize and sustain you. Rest assured, you do not need to become the poster person for cancer if being on stage for something as private as your health is not of interest.

Control your role
Additionally, take time to get clear about which stages you enjoy and which you want to avoid. For example, you may love being "on" for work, but hate being so accessible when it comes to your private life, or more specifically your health. You may be thinking, "I do not want to be the star in the cancer show." You will likely want to serve as your own agent, control your role, and decide which aspects of visibility and sharing you want to own, delegate, or decline.

Plan your milestones
Milestones may be a big deal to you because they help you measure your success. What milestones are important to you? What key markers will be meaningful for measuring your progress? Something that has worked for someone else might not mean much to you, so find the thing that you can really get behind. Ringing the bell at the end of a chemotherapy or radiation regimen is a tradition in many cancer centers. You may be the type of person who not only wants to ring the bell, but also make sure people see you doing it! That's great; it will help sustain you. You naturally know that you're inspiring and educating people by allowing them in on your cancer journey. Let yourself shine.

Be independent
Independence and autonomy are important to people with this strength. Is there anything you'd like to do by yourself? You may love having your partner or a close friend take you to chemotherapy. But you may decide to venture out to a support group, a wig fitting, or an oncology

appointment by yourself. People naturally worry about you feeling lonely during your treatment but reassure them you appreciate the support and are energized by doing some things on your own.

Seek input on the best

Prior to your cancer diagnosis, you were likely selective with the sources of information you consumed and the individuals you sought for advice. If your type of cancer is common with an abundant amount of information, ask your care team, "What are the best cancer materials I should read? What other institutions or organizations do you consider to be elite and cream of the crop? What resources would you avoid?" Your discernment of wanting only the best can be a great advantage for where you're spending your time and energy.

Consider opportunities to give back

You have an internal fire which leads you to be bold, brave, and courageous. This intensity can be used for cancer-related efforts. There are so many opportunities to give back to the cancer community. Are you motivated to help with any causes that aid in cancer prevention, research, treatment, or recovery? Many survivors work to build awareness, raise funds, encourage health screenings, mentor those newly diagnosed, or engage in advocacy work. Dr. Bonaminio said she is very open about sharing her journey, explains the value of 3D mammograms to friends and colleagues, and is a champion to others for screening. Additionally, she was asked to deliver the University of Kansas School of Medicine graduation speech in 2022 and described her leadership style as "that of consequential leadership, including conviction, courage, composure, communication, and compassion." Those are powerful qualities for a leader like Dr. Bonaminio, with her Significance strength.

The opportunities for this strength in advocacy are endless including influencing policy change, promoting cancer research, or addressing health disparities and fighting for health equity. The American Cancer Society Cancer Action Network, ACS CAN, is an example of a nonprofit and nonpartisan advocacy group.[72] "With the help of volunteers, ACS CAN campaigns have led to 35 states going smoke-free and increased federal cancer research funding for the National Institute of Health." If advocacy work piques your curiosity, learn more from people and organizations aligned with your interests or frustrations related to cancer.

Cancer Cautions

Connect small steps to the larger goal
You may dread boring and mundane tasks—they don't feel significant or exceptional. If your treatment plan includes dozens of chemotherapy or radiation sessions, these may quickly become monotonous. Connect these small steps to the larger outcome. Remind yourself that each chemo infusion, radiation session, physical therapy appointment, and counseling session are all steps toward your overall health goal. It will help you to mentally connect each individual step to the larger, incredible goal and outcome you desire. Consider making a scoreboard or display where you can celebrate crossing off each task, like a blood draw, chemo session, or MRI, so that you can visually see and track your progress.

Ensure your need to be seen is met
You may crave feedback and recognition. Some care providers are more focused on your cancer than you as an individual. This disconnect could make you feel invisible and like just another cancer patient. Ask questions to better understand what makes your case unique. If you still don't feel seen, consider switching healthcare providers while evaluating the time and cost of making that move. If you are looking for more empathy, attention, or feedback regarding your treatment and progress, consider a referral to a psychologist or therapist where you are the primary focus. It's important to get your needs met so that this strength can help sustain you.

---

72 American Cancer Society, Cancer Action Network (ACS CAN). Available at: https://www.cancer.org/involved/volunteer/acs-can.html.

You don't have to make cancer your legacy

Cancer does not have to be part of your legacy. You may not want to be involved in the cancer arena during or after your treatment. You may view this part of your life as a bump in the road, blip on the radar, or small chapter of your memoir. On your life resume, cancer survivor can be a footnote at the end rather than the header. Do not feel obligated or pressured to infuse cancer into your aspirations. You don't owe cancer anything.

Strategic

People exceptionally talented in the Strategic theme quickly spot patterns and issues that others miss. They generate alternative paths forward and choose the most effective one.

You have the natural ability to sort through clutter and find the best way forward. This distinct way of thinking cannot be taught. You see patterns where others see complexity. Mindful of these patterns, you play out alternative scenarios, always asking, "What if this happened? OK, then what if this happened?" This recurring question helps you visualize and evaluate potential obstacles and possibilities. Guided by where you see each path leading, you start to make selections. You discard the paths that lead nowhere. You discard the paths that lead straight into resistance. You discard the paths that lead into a fog of confusion. You continually assess and make selections until you arrive at your chosen path—your strategy.

You're taking something extraordinarily complex and making it very simple, putting key milestones in place, and asking a lot of questions. What you did by taking me through this strengths assessment helped me recognize that I'm actually leaning on my greatest strength.

—Holly, breast cancer survivor

Characteristics of Those with Strategic Talents

Creative	Option-aware	Future-oriented
Selective	Insightful	Clear
Intuitive	Anticipating	Thoughtful

Cancer Connection

People with Strategic as a strength can see the big picture, consider a variety of options, and create a plan. A cancer diagnosis certainly sets you up to use this strength. Your brain naturally sees things in a series of phases, stages, changes, and transitions. Many types of cancer follow this sort of pattern. Some cancer survivors have a hard time grasping the length of their treatment plan, which may extend many months or even years, and can get discouraged. Others may find themselves deep in the details or minutiae of one small part of their treatment and get overwhelmed. Your Strategic strength will help you avoid these pitfalls because you can naturally zoom out and see the larger plan.

Give yourself time to think, ponder the possibilities, and develop plans that will help you with your treatment and healing process. As you are in the beginning stage of evaluating your options, it might be helpful for you to write or draw the plans you are considering. You may need to set time on your calendar or change your typical routines to allow time for effective treatment planning sessions. Strategic is one of the more common of the 34 CliftonStrengths, so you may have friends or colleagues you can partner with for strategizing. Who do you know who can draw up a plan on the back of a napkin or a whiteboard? These thought partners do not have to be cancer survivors or even have experience with healthcare or medical challenges. You both will be energized by evaluating different options, patterns, and potential scenarios. If you're uncomfortable working through this process with people you know, consider engaging a therapist or trusted resource to help you instead.

As you continue through your cancer experience, remember your Strategic strength makes it easy for you to quickly envision plans, and family and friends may need you to describe how you came to your decision. You may need to explain your thinking even though your choices feel obvious to you. These people are most likely not questioning your judgment but can't connect the dots as clearly as you do. Bring them up to speed so they can support you, execute your plans, and share as needed with others on your care team. Trust me—I am one of these people. Strategic is number 34 on my list of CliftonStrengths—dead last. I love being around thought leaders with this strength because once they explain their plan and how they made their decision, I get it and can get moving on bringing their vision to life. Buy-in matters.

Cancer Considerations

Lean into the complexity
The shock of the diagnosis coupled with all the decisions to be made is overwhelming for most. It can feel like a puzzle without corners and like there's not a single right or clear path. With your Strategic strength, you are exceptional at quickly considering and analyzing all your options. You've likely experienced times in your life when others were overwhelmed by a complex project, and you were easily able to guide them through the maze to a strong finish. You can do that for yourself now.

We met Holly LaVallie in Part One of this book. She was a vice president in marketing with a demanding leadership role and a single mom raising two teenage daughters when she received her breast cancer diagnosis. She quickly shifted into project planning mode, evaluated all her options, made swift decisions, and got into treatment at Mayo Clinic in Rochester, Minnesota. I interviewed Holly for a strength series I was doing during Breast Cancer Awareness Month.[73] The way she described how she approached her diagnosis and, later, learned about her top

---

73 McCausland, T., *Follow Your Strengths*, (2021). "Strategic: Holly LaVallie." Available at: https://www.followyourstrengths.com/blog/achiever-jen-slabas-guidi-9msly-tw2p2-4llj7.

strength of Strategic, is incredible. If you listen to the interview on my website I say, "If you have a mic, why don't you go ahead and drop it." I talked about this in Part One but it's worth repeating. Here is what she shared during this mic drop moment:

> As I was going through my diagnosis, so many people said, "Where are your emotions? Why are you being so pragmatic?" I started to wonder if maybe I was stuffing my emotions down. But when I took the CliftonStrengths assessment, it provided this incredible light for me. I realized, no Holly, you are not stuffing things down. How you're handling the hardest thing you've been through is by leaning into your greatest strength and you didn't even know that you're doing it. You're taking something extraordinarily complex and making it very simple, putting key milestones in place, and asking a lot of questions. The other part I learned from taking the assessment is that people with the Strategic strength go through all the potential outcomes, good and bad, and they weigh them out to find a range of risk, the highest upside and the lowest downside. When I very naturally did that with my diagnosis, I found out my risk is manageable. Now it's just a matter of managing it. I'm actually quite grateful because I thought I was stuffing some emotions. What you did by taking me through this strength assessment helped me recognize that I'm actually leaning on my greatest strength.

Manage change effortlessly
Managing change is part of having a serious health condition and navigating the healthcare arena. You will undoubtedly face disruptions and delays during your cancer experience. Use your Strategic strength to switch gears, consider a new or evolving option, and move forward with your best revised plan. Remind yourself that change is part of your treatment plan, and you are excellent at navigating it. This natural ability of yours to move nearly effortlessly through disruption and change will help

you conserve energy, reduce stress, and adjust your care as new information arises.

Make a support plan
If you plan to take a leave of absence from work or reduce your hours scheduled, create a high-level plan of how that could look and recruit others to help execute your vision. Design your ideal plan for the additional support you'd like to have at home with projects, food prep, or yardwork. While you create the outline of your request, such as three weeknight dinners for your family per week, your supporters can handle the details of designing the menu and creating the schedule for food drop-offs. If you feel bogged down in minor details, share this concern with your colleagues or supporters and ask for help with the tasks that feel draining.

Cancer Cautions

Bring people along with you
You are naturally a quick thinker and may see the path forward more easily or earlier than some of your supporters. You may sense they are a couple of steps behind you in digesting and processing your cancer diagnosis, treatment plan, or other life impacts. It will help them if you can briefly explain your thought process, the possibilities you considered, the ones you discarded, and how you landed on your decision. This conversation could be related to anything from your decision to continue working full time, why you selected one care center over another, or your plan on how to communicate your health updates.

Beware of wasting energy on the small stuff
You are not a fan of people or organizations doing things the way they have always been done. You could become frustrated with your medical care if you sense inefficiencies or a lack of innovation, or endure a poor patient experience. For example, you may not be satisfied with the

answers you receive when you question the registration and scheduling process in one department. Ask yourself if this is an area that is negatively impacting your overall care and if you want to spend your energy digging into this concern. Keep your eye on the big picture.

Woo

People exceptionally talented in the Woo theme love meeting new people and winning them over. They enjoy socializing and making connections.

Woo stands for winning others over. You enjoy the challenge of meeting new people and getting them to like you. Strangers rarely intimidate you. On the contrary, strangers can be energizing. You are drawn to them. You want to learn their names, ask them questions and find areas of common interest so you can build rapport. Some people shy away from initiating conversations because they worry about running out of things to say. You don't. Not only are you rarely at a loss for words, but you love introducing yourself and making a connection. Once the connection is made, you are quite happy to move on. There are new people to meet, new rooms to work, new crowds to mingle in. In your world, there are no strangers, only friends you haven't met yet—lots of them.

I took the time to get to know the staff at the cancer center. I made it a point to know their names and ask questions about them.

—*Erica, breast cancer survivor*

Characteristics of Those with Woo Talents

Charming	Socially proactive	Outgoing
Engaging	Winsome	Interactive
Influential	Gregarious	Initiating
Socially energetic		

Cancer Connection

People with Woo are social magnets. They are drawn to people, and people are typically drawn to them. Some strengths are more challenging to observe than others, but not Woo. People with this strength have an incredible gift for gab and can create comfort and warmth in any room that is easy to see and hear. They are intentional with creating memorable first impressions by how they welcome and greet others and how they create connection.

When it comes to your cancer diagnosis, you will still need people and they will still need you. If your care plan impacts your daily routine, make sure that people you can woo, and be wooed by, are part of your new schedule. You may need to work remotely, take a leave of absence, or travel less for your job. Your exercise schedule may shift from hot yoga classes inside with a group to walking outside with a friend or working 1:1 with a personal trainer to protect your immune system. Regardless of what changes, people need to be part of it. Will you get to see new people at a coffee shop, walking your dog outside, or through reconnecting with old friends on a video conference? Even short, casual interactions will boost your energy. Keep in mind that by filling your own gas tank with this social energy, you are also undoubtedly filling the tanks of others too.

Woo falls in the Influencing domain. You make an impact on each person you meet, and this can make a huge difference in the lives of many due to the ripple effect of your presence. Think about how you want to leverage your Woo strength as you move through your cancer experience.

Give thought to your current network, your potential growing network, and your life goals. It doesn't have to be related to cancer but continue to gain clarity on the difference you want to make in people's lives through the energy and connections you so naturally create.

Cancer Considerations

You will bring light
With your strength of meeting new people and creating immediate connections, you can quickly set the tone of initial meetings with your doctor and care team members which will uplift them and you. You are probably a natural at learning peoples' names and referring to them by name in the future. If that's something that is important to you, consider carrying a small notepad or an electronic option for taking "Name Notes." You will also interact with countless people from the time you walk through the doors of the hospital or treatment center—from the registration clerk to the patient and caregiver sitting next to you in the waiting room. Your sincere smile, your ease with words, and your personable style may be just what they need to positively impact their day. Erica, a cancer survivor with the Woo strength shared, "I took the time to get to know the staff at the cancer center. I made it a point to know their names and ask questions about them. This helped me feel connected but also allowed me to see and remember that they were people, and they have hard days too. I think this intentional connecting ultimately helped me not feel sorry for myself too." Be sure to read the room on how much interaction people are open to, but do not hold back on your charming and comforting way. It may be the one bright light in an otherwise darker day for a patient or provider.

Share significant milestones
Consider incorporating a celebration into one of your key milestones, such as completing chemotherapy or radiation treatments. Some cancer survivors enjoy celebrating the anniversary of their diagnosis, surgery, or

the day they heard the words "No Evidence of Disease," or NED. If these dates on the calendar are significant to you, share this with your network of friends and family and invite them to join the party. They will expect nothing less from their loved one with Woo and will absolutely love joining in the social joy with you.

What can you make fun?

People with the Woo strength are often associated with fun. They have a special spark about them and can effortlessly create energy wherever they go. Granted, the words cancer and fun don't typically go together, but is there any way you can infuse some fun energy into this experience? This could include the people you invite to join you for appointments or the activities or discussions that occupy your time in the waiting rooms. Contrary to what people might envision, cancer centers are sometimes filled with card games, group pictures, matching t-shirts, and laughter.

I met Michelle at the Gallup Strengths Summit in Omaha in 2018. She reached out to me after hearing my podcast interview with host Jim Collison on Gallup's *Called to Coach*.[74] Our cancer journeys were eerily similar as we were diagnosed within 10 days of one another. Michelle has Woo and shared some incredible examples of how she incorporated fun into her cancer experience. She put her marketing expertise to use by creating a theme of Fighting Mich's Tumor with Humor which was a perfect slogan for t-shirts worn by her supporters. She also shared, "I truly believe the positive outcome of this journey has been a result of what I like to call the Four F's—Faith, Family, Friends, and always keeping things FUN!" Michelle was working at Southwest Airlines during her treatment, and her team turned their annual Texas State Fair outing into a breast cancer themed day called "Wiggin' Out." Her team members embraced this theme and wore pink, along with a wig, which meant so much to Michelle. She shared, "What a great way to get my mind off all the upcoming procedures and surgeries. I am so blessed."

---

74 *Called to Coach* podcast with Jim Collison, "Facing a Life Crisis with the Help of Strengths." Available at: https://www.gallup.com/cliftonstrengths/en/249761/facing-life-crisis-help-strengths.aspx.

Handling introductions to the newly diagnosed

As you continue to progress through the months and years of being a cancer survivor, people will naturally reach out to you with questions or to see if they can introduce you to somebody newly diagnosed. Think about how you'd like to respond to these requests. You may enjoy connecting with new people and serving as a mentor. If not, that's okay too. Refer them to other helpful resources or people or tell them you need your energy for healing. If you feel inspired, you could create a brief document with your thoughts, advice, and any resources related to your type of cancer. Sarah, a breast cancer survivor with a large network, created a Facebook Messenger group chat for newly diagnosed friends and acquaintances. She encouraged people to ask any questions, and complete strangers from the group would quickly respond. This blew me away the night of my diagnosis as I posted a simple question in the chat asking how people made the decision on what cancer center to select. I went to bed that night shortly after making that post, and when I woke up, all eight women in the group had responded. The group quadrupled in size in just a few years and is an example of the exponential power of the Woo strength.

Use your network for good

If the political arena of healthcare or cancer excites you, your vast network could support you in championing a particular cause. What do you want to see happen and who do you know who can help? Leverage your network to speed toward outcomes that will help cancer patients, research, and prevention efforts. Siddhartha Mukherjee, author of the Pulitzer Prize–winning book *The Emperor of All Maladies: A Biography of Cancer*,[75] says of Mary Woodard Lasker:[76]

---

75   Mukherjee, Siddhartha (2010). *The Emperor of All Maladies: A Biography of Cancer*, Scribner.

76   Lasker Foundation, "Empress of All Maladies: Mary Lasker." Available at: https://laskerfoundation.org/empress-of-all-maladies-mary-lasker.

. . . a powerful businesswoman, art dealer, and philanthropist who led a crusade to win passage of the National Cancer Act in 1971 and to dramatically increase funding for the National Institute of Health. As she often reminded Congress, "If you think research is expensive, try disease."

He said, too, "Mary Lasker was an entrepreneur; she was a socialite. She was kind of a legendary networker." The Lasker Foundation President added, "She leveraged her networks in the media, Madison Avenue, Hollywood, Capitol Hill and the citadels of academia to build partnerships that could move the needle in Congress and in the Oval Office." Although Mary Lasker passed away at the age of 93 in 1993 and did not take Gallup's CliftonStrengths assessment, my prediction is she would definitely have had Woo high on her list. Never underestimate what a difference you can make with this strength.

Cancer Cautions

Honor your desire for privacy
Although you know a lot of people, it doesn't mean they need to be informed of your diagnosis and medical updates if you don't want them to. Even if you're typically an open book, you may prefer to keep this chapter private or limited to your invite-only book club, so to speak.

Explain how your Woo strength helps you
If you approach your cancer experience the way you approach life, some people may express concern, worry that you are in denial, performing a positivity show, or refusing to accept that this is a serious situation. While you don't need to justify your approach, be prepared for this feedback and give some thought to how you will handle your concerned or intrusive supporters.

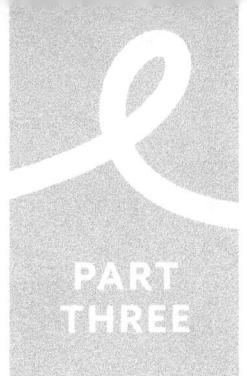

PART THREE

CAREGIVER CONSIDERATIONS

My house is a hive of people trying to save my life by doing errands. There is everything to do and nothing to be done.

—*Dr. Kate Bowler, Professor of Religious History at Duke University and colon cancer survivor*

Introduction

Caring for a loved one with a cancer diagnosis can be difficult, overwhelming, and emotionally draining. It can also build a deeper connection and be a rewarding experience. You will be there in so many ways, from going to oncology appointments and picking up prescriptions, to making dinner and sitting with them when they're sick. Caregivers often wonder how to best support and help their loved one with cancer. Paying attention to the way they think, feel, and behave is a helpful strategy for you to deliver the best support based on their specific needs. Understanding their strengths and asking strengths-based questions will change how you give support and may end up drawing you much closer together.

As noted in Part One, there is good reason to help cancer patients focus on their strengths as it leads to improved health and wellness outcomes. While they will undoubtedly face challenges and setbacks, they will also encounter positive events and emotions along the way. Dr. Clifton's teachings encouraged us to focus on what is strong instead of obsessing over what is wrong. Although that advice is easier to follow when life is relatively stable, it doesn't mean we should ignore it during a health crisis. As a caretaker, encourage your loved one to take note of areas in their life that are going well. Additionally, challenge them to reflect on how they handled adversity effectively in the past. Gallup's book *CliftonStrengths for Students* explains that, "Helping others recognize the strength they have demonstrated in the past can give them hope and confidence now and in the future."[77]

---

77   https://www.followyourstrengths.com/book.

Some of you are caring for a parent, child, partner, sibling, or close friend. You may have a front row seat in observing how this diagnosis impacts their daily life, routines, energy levels, and emotions. Be sure not to underestimate the impact it may have on your daily life as well. There are great caregiver resources available from organizations like the American Cancer Society, the National Cancer Institute, therapists, and possibly through your work Employee Assistance Program, if applicable. Caregiver support resources are listed in the Resources for Surviving Cancer with Your Strengths section for this book as well. You may also want to consider attending a support group or reaching out to others who have been caregivers.

A friend of mine and a Gallup-Certified Strengths Coach, Anna Krueger, has a deeply personal experience serving as caregiver for her mom, Sharon. She has some advice to share on how to approach your role as caregiver by honoring the strengths of your loved one while also tending to your own strengths, health, and well-being.

> My mom, Sharon Grammer, was a true shining light in the cancer community. She was diagnosed with Stage 4 cancer and expected to live for three months, but she ended up living for 11 years. As her caregiver, I was able to witness up close how she used her strengths to keep her emotional tank full while navigating her cancer experience. Some of her top strengths were Empathy, Communication, Connectedness, Woo, Belief and Positivity. Because of her natural desire to uplift others, she started a nonprofit for cancer patients to encourage them on their first day of chemotherapy. Mom delivered a gift bag with 14 wrapped gifts inside—enough to open one a day for two weeks after their first chemo treatment. She also included a letter inviting them to call her anytime. By the time she passed, over 3,000 gift bags had been delivered. Without a doubt, I know this nonprofit fed her strengths and fueled her desire to live and make a difference.
>
> By paying close attention to my mom's strengths, I knew that collecting meaningful words spoken to my mom would

uplift her spirit. For example, I asked her friends to send cards of encouragement. I collected them and delivered them to her on a random day, simply to uplift her. Another time I made a 3-ring binder with printouts of social posts and comments that praised my mom for the difference she was making in people's lives. These items became some of her favorite possessions.

As her caregiver, I learned to pay attention to what I needed, as well. When caregiving, so much energy and attention is directed to the cancer patient—which is needed—yet it can leave you feeling depleted and drained if you are not intentional about also caring for yourself. I have high Empathy and Positivity, and during my caregiving years I had to shield myself from hearing negative things outside of mom's cancer diagnosis. For me, this meant deleting news apps off my phone, avoiding people that were generally negative by nature, and unfollowing certain social accounts. My high Adaptability and Connectedness strengths are energized by spending time in nature, and my Communication strength needs to verbally process events for them to feel real. I became more intentional about spending time in beautiful places—by the lake, in the mountains—and while there, I would take time to journal my thoughts. My Empathy and Positivity strengths were aware of the impact my venting may have on others around me, so writing became the safe space for me to feel and share what was on my heart.

The love and connection between Anna and her mother is evident in the stories she shares about her and the profound impact her nonprofit made in the lives of others. As you provide caregiving support for your loved one, please keep Anna's experience in mind. Understanding her mom's strengths allowed her to customize the support and recognition she provided. As you pour so much of your time, energy, and heart into helping your loved one through their cancer experience, be sure you are receiving appropriate love and care as well. If you would like to understand your strengths further and begin thinking about how to use your natural talents in a caregiving role or beyond, please visit the How to Discover Your Strengths section of the book in Part One to learn how to complete the CliftonStrengths assessment or other strengths-based exercises.

Achiever

Your loved one with Achiever talents may be operating on less energy; however, their instinct will still be to complete and finish things. Honor this. It may feel like they are pushing too hard, but accomplishing activities, tasks, or projects may strengthen their spirit rather than deplete their energy. Common advice for many cancer patients includes slowing down and resting. While that is generally good advice, it is not always the best advice for those with Achiever talents, given their natural drive toward productivity.

Consider areas where you can help them get things done. For example, what could they finish while they sit in the waiting rooms before appointments? If they have certain days between treatments where they feel better than others, what can you help ensure they accomplish? People with Achiever talents will be energized by your support in moving things toward completion. Look for tasks you can help them complete and be sure to help them celebrate! For example, celebrate the halfway point of chemo completions, celebrate when major care decisions are made, or celebrate anniversaries of having No Evidence of Disease (NED).

Ask your loved one these questions
- What did you get done this week?
- Are there any tasks, like folding laundry, mowing the lawn, or watering flowers, you'd like to check off your list? Can I help?
- What were you hoping to get done this week, but couldn't? What can I help you finish?
- What is something that would make you feel so good to have done?
- How can we celebrate what you've accomplished? What feels best to you?

Activator

Your loved one with Activator talents may be operating on less energy; however, their instinct will still be to start or initiate projects and plans. Honor this. It may feel like they are pushing too hard, but seeing things move forward will increase their energy.

Patients with the Activator strength may tire of the routine involved in doctor's appointments, blood draws, chemo, or radiation. If you're accompanying them, suggest something new. Perhaps it's as simple as a time-passing activity in the waiting rooms. I saw one patient playing cribbage each visit while waiting to see the doctor. Four people sat around a table in the waiting room and passed the time with a fun game of cards. Consider checking out a new restaurant or place for a healthy snack before or after treatment, depending on their appetite and energy. Variety and the feeling of a new beginning may be invigorating.

It is common for cancer patients to celebrate the final milestones during various phases of treatment. For example, some cancer centers and hospitals have a bell for patients to ring after they complete their final chemotherapy or radiation treatment. Keep in mind that people with Activator talents thrive when starting or initiating action and progress. In addition to those traditional celebrations commonly reserved for completing phases of treatment, consider celebrating the beginning of these phases as this is where people with Activator talents are typically strongest.

Ask your loved one these questions
- What can I help you start? Do you need me to help you research any cancer topics or products?

- Is there anything you're avoiding, like paperwork or picking up prescriptions, that I can help move forward?
- Are there any tasks or decisions that have slowed or stalled that you'd like to move forward? How can I help create some movement and traction?
- What can I help you do now instead of later? For example, can I be proactive and finish a house project early so you don't have to worry about it during your surgery recovery?
- What can we make progress on today? Point me in the right direction, and I'll get things started.

Adaptability

Your loved one with the Adaptability strength is brilliant with NOW and TODAY and will seem grounded and present each day beyond their diagnosis. While for many of us, this approach may be mind-boggling, please keep in mind their instinct is to remain calm and flexible even when life gets tough and scary. Honor this. It may even appear as denial or naivety to you, but responding to challenges and pressures during the day may boost their energy.

Patients with Adaptability talents can go with the flow and adapt quickly to change. If that is not easy for you, be sure to follow their lead. For example, navigating the healthcare system schedule, treatments, or logistics may frustrate you. If you're helping them with scheduling or accompanying them to appointments, do not impose your frustration. They may see the waiting room or schedule changes simply as part of the deal and not be upset. You are supporting them, so work to manage your emotions if your own frustration or anger arises. Take a walk, do some deep breathing, talk to the nurse out of their earshot. The last thing you want to do is drain their energy based on your concerns. Their healthcare experience should be patient-centered, so do your best to allow their incredible strength of flexibility to shine. Take note of it. Respect it. Recognize it. Praise it. Be specific about what you're noticing and how you're impressed with their ability to adapt, respond, and be gracious during the midst of change and challenges in their cancer journey.

Ask your loved one these questions
- How are you feeling today and what would make you feel even better?

- Is there anything spontaneous that sounds good to do soon?
- Would you like to shift gears and change our original plan for the day?
- Are there any upcoming tests, procedures, or appointments you need to prepare for? How can I help you with researching, getting organized, or preparing in advance?

Analytical

Your loved one with Analytical talents will handle a cancer diagnosis differently than most. While many patients are rattled and emotional, people with this strength tend to be calm, logical, and serious. You may need to relay this to others who care about them including family, friends, and colleagues. People may view their reaction to this diagnosis as concerning if they don't show much emotion, and some may even suspect they are depressed or in denial. If possible, reassure supporters that they are approaching the diagnosis and decision-making process rationally and objectively.

Don't make assumptions about how they are feeling. Ask them to share their feelings with you. Be clear and direct with your questions and listen carefully to their requests and desires. Cancer can be a very emotional life event, but your loved one may prefer a calmer, more grounded approach to the experience. Make sure you are following their lead on what is most helpful to them rather than what you've observed as helpful to other cancer survivors.

Ask your loved one these questions
- Is there any data or information you're curious about or missing? Can I help research anything for you?
- I know you want to have all the facts before making decisions and you typically don't rush into action. If there are timelines we need to meet, what would help you come to a final decision and act? Do you want somebody to brainstorm with, play out different scenarios, or simply give you a deadline?

- Do you have physical or electronic articles, research, or ideas you're exploring? What can I do to help you create a system for the answers to your questions?
- How are you feeling about the mental and emotional side of cancer? Do you want to talk about it with me, another cancer survivor, or a professional?
- Is anything annoying you right now from caring supporters? For example, people may be trying to make t-shirts in your honor or organizing a meal train. If those things make you cringe and feel worse, I can help reroute those with good intentions.

Arranger

Your loved one with the Arranger strength is likely comfortable coordinating their healthcare plans and related activities. Many people may admire their ability to have so many things going on simultaneously. Their instinct is to thrive in dynamic, complex environments, so honor this. It may even appear as them taking on too much needlessly to you, but having numerous "balls in the air," so to speak, may give them a much-needed energy boost.

Patients with Arranger talents can navigate change and adjust accordingly. In fact, they are often the ones who are driving the change. They may have a care center, surgeon, and surgery confirmed. Then, after gathering more information, decide to change centers, surgeons, and types of surgeries! They will also quickly adjust to schedule changes, new members of their care team, or treatment side effects. You may feel anxious or annoyed when their medical plan veers off the path. Pay close attention to their response though as they may not even be fazed. Let them know you're impressed with how quickly they can shift gears and move forward on their new path.

Ask your loved one these questions
- What would make today's plan run more smoothly? How can I help make that happen?
- If you could juggle one more thing in your schedule right now, what would that one thing be? Would you like to juggle it yourself or outsource it to somebody else?

- If it feels like you are juggling too many things, what can be removed? Do you need somebody else to handle it or is it something that can be taken off your plate entirely?
- Is there anyone who has information or a skillset that could help you with something, either at work or at home? Can I reach out to them for help?
- What would the ideal schedule be for your treatment days? What flexibility would you like to build into the plan?
- Would you like to change our original plan for the day? For the week?

Belief

Your loved one with the Belief strength may be operating on less energy; however, their instinct will still be to serve others. Honor this. It may feel like they are being too altruistic given their current health crisis, but focusing on an important cause or mission may be energizing to them.

Common advice for many cancer patients includes something along the lines of making yourself a priority. While that generally isn't bad advice for cancer patients, it may not sit well for those with Belief talents, given their natural mindset of helping and serving others. They take their core values, commitments, and responsibilities very seriously. It may be helpful if you can encourage them in both arenas—their priorities beyond cancer and their health and well-being.

Consider areas where you can help them fulfill their mission or purpose. For example, is there a cause or an organization they actively support? Are there any tasks that you can help them complete while in waiting rooms, during chemo treatments, or on days they are resting at home? People with the Belief strength will be energized by your support in helping them continue to make a difference.

Ask your loved one these questions
- What are some of your core values you want to make sure we stick to during your cancer experience? For example, family, inner peace, or fun may be things you value in your life. What can we do to make sure your life still reflects those values, even during this time of adversity?

- What causes are currently most important to you? What type of involvement do you think you can maintain during your treatment and healing?
- Is there anything you feel strongly about that you'd like your supporters to understand about cancer or your treatment plan? How can I help to convey that message? For example, you may feel strongly that you do not want people to raise money on your behalf but would prefer they donate to the local cancer clinic instead.
- Are there family members or close friends who you would like to spend more time with during your cancer experience? I know they mean so much to you, so please let me know how I can best help coordinate time or activities together, as your energy allows.

Command

Your loved one with the Command strength has likely been known as a leader and somebody others have looked to for guidance and direction. Even now, in a vulnerable position because of their health scare, that doesn't mean they can't still lead. Look to them to set the direction before you offer up ideas. They will probably set the tone for their cancer experience anyway but work on asking them good questions and reminding them of their natural leadership presence and strength if you sense any hesitation or doubt.

You are used to your person being a confident decision-maker. Cancer won't take that strength away from them, but the process could look different. They will probably need more information, time, or conversations than usual to reach clarity on their decisions. If this seems to frustrate them, it may help for you to reassure them of their strength and remind them that this is new territory.

Ask your loved one these questions
- What is your gut telling you about the decisions you face? Are we missing information or is there anything unclear to you? Who do we need to ask?
- What tension or apprehension are you sensing within yourself or those close to you? What are some things we can do to increase trust, confidence, and clarity?
- What do you think is best to do next? Can I or anyone else help with it?
- Are you comfortable with your care team? How do you feel they are doing with guiding your treatment plan?
- What support do you need from others? What do you want us to do to help?

Communication

Your loved one with the Communication strength has likely always had a way with words. As they navigate their cancer diagnosis and treatment plan, this strength may come out in a variety of ways. They may be interested in talking with other cancer survivors through 1:1 conversations or support groups. Some people with this strength say that an experience doesn't feel like it really happened until they get a chance to talk about it. So they may need more time to process through their cancer diagnosis, procedures, and emotions with family, friends, or a trained professional. Words are important to them, so they may be driven to control the narrative and make sure people understand the correct vocabulary and outlook for their diagnosis and path forward. Pay close attention to what they say and use the same words they use. It's also very likely they may NOT want to talk through their feelings. They may prefer spending time writing, journaling, or developing stories in their head. Let them be in the driver's seat of their communication plan, so to speak, and things will be all right.

People with Communication talents are great at bringing everyday moments to life through their words and expressions. They may be known as funny, entertaining, great storytellers, or as skilled conversationalists. Consider ways you can support them in processing this experience, sharing as they wish, and preserving any documents, pictures, gifts, or mementos for remembrance along the way. It's difficult to predict how people will process a cancer diagnosis and steps of their treatment plan. Let them take the lead on setting the mood for doctor's visits and conversations about their health. You may anticipate somber visits to the oncologist, yet they may walk out of the hospital joking about an experience in the waiting room.

Ask your loved one these questions
- What key points do you want people to know about your cancer? What are the exact words we should use? Are there any words we should avoid using? For example, I never use the word *remission* to describe my health. My care team has said there is *No Evidence of Disease* (NED) and that is my preferred terminology.
- What do you and don't you want to talk about? Would you like for me to share my thoughts or just listen?
- When we get together with a group of friends, are there updates you want to share? Are there any details you'd prefer we keep private?
- How can I help you capture your thoughts, questions, and stories about this experience?
- Can I help contact anyone to arrange time for you to connect with over coffee, lunch, or a phone call?

Competition

Your loved one with the strength of Competition will instinctively find ways to measure, compare, push, and win. This isn't going to change because of their diagnosis. It may feel like they are pushing too hard from your perspective, but having benchmarks and goals related to their treatment plan may help fuel their internal fire.

Patients with Competition talents may be bored by the routine involved in doctor's appointments and treatments if there is no new benchmark for them to beat. If you're accompanying them, suggest something where they can win while they wait. Perhaps it's a new card game, a board game, or a word game played in the waiting room. Consider challenging them with a goal to complete during chemo. For example, if they would like to stay awake during treatment, challenge them to read 15 pages in their book or to write five thank-you notes to supporters. Having a measure for success will serve as a productive distraction.

One thing to note about the Competition strength is the external awareness it brings. Do not assume that all wins are created equal. Your loved one may not care if they beat a personal record. They want to win against others who are brave enough to be in the arena too. When your person does not feel they are set up to perform well, they may withdraw and not even want to compete. Rather than encouraging them to look at how far they've come, consider sharing an externally motivated challenge, like what they might be interested in competing for next, or how they would like to approach things differently on the next round of treatment.

Many people with Competition talents enjoy public recognition. Verify if this is the case for your loved one. Is there a way to celebrate a cancer milestone? For example, if they receive a positive report from a scan or a blood draw, how can you create a way to help them feel seen? If their tumors are shrinking, what type of high five or fist bump would help them celebrate? It is common for cancer patients to celebrate the final milestones during various phases of treatment. You know that bell patients ring after they complete their final chemotherapy or radiation treatment? People with Competition talents thrive when measuring and winning. Even if they're exhausted and don't feel up for this tradition, encourage them to ring that bell. Celebrate loudly and with photos.

Ask your loved one these questions
- What does a win look like for you today? How can I help?
- What health-related metrics or milestones do you want to visibly track? Is there a way I can help you create a scoreboard?
- What is something you're currently measuring? How could we move the needle together?
- Who do you consider a winner? Can I help track down resources about them or facilitate a conversation? Being with other winners will give you a boost.

Connectedness

Your loved one with Connectedness talents is intuitive and easily sees connections between people, places, and events. They may focus more on understanding their treatment plan options than understanding the cause of their cancer. Follow their lead on this, despite your own potential curiosity to know more about the diagnosis. They have a natural ability to zoom out from the details and are great at seeing the big picture in situations. Trust what they share with you, even if you haven't connected all those dots yet. As you express your trust, it's fine to ask questions about how they are making these connections as long as you come from a place of curiosity versus disbelief or judgment.

While your person's intuitive nature and big picture thinking are definite strengths, they may feel overwhelmed by the sheer vastness of cancer's reach, impacting millions around the world. It may be helpful for you to help them zoom in and focus on what's right in front of them from time to time. Remind them to "Think global, and act local," just as Mary Sue, a cancer survivor with the strength of Connectedness, shared in Part Two.

Ask your loved one these questions
- What connections are you seeing or feeling during your cancer experience? Are you noticing anything across the people, places, or events you're experiencing?
- Is there any place you feel confused about your options or unable to put together information in a way that makes sense to you about your treatment plan? What information can I help you gather or what questions can I help you ask at your upcoming appointments?

- Would you like to incorporate more nature into your life, even in small ways like short walks, taking a day trip to the lake, or framing pictures of flowers or wildlife? How can I help with anything?
- I know you value humanity on a global scale and big picture thinking. Has your health experience brought any new ideas or insights to you? What expanded thinking have you been doing, and would it be helpful to share your thoughts with anyone?

Consistency

Your loved one with Consistency talents has had their predictable world rocked by their cancer diagnosis. They will need ways to maintain routines, steadiness, and balance in their lives. Help brainstorm ways you can help them create this sense of calm and clarity, despite cancer creating a huge detour on their daily schedule. Have conversations with them about how you can best help to support their desired exercise, nutrition, sleep, or medical appointment routines.

Additionally, people with this strength value fairness and equality. They may not ask for any extra attention or special treatment as they move through their cancer experience. There are things that they may really want and need but hesitate to ask for as they don't want to be perceived as getting special treatment. Be aware of this and ask what they need since they may not initiate the request. Following doctor's orders will be automatic for your loved one, and you will likely witness an ideal patient in action since they tend to thrive in situations with clear rules and expectations. Not many people are excited about SOP's, or Standard Operating Procedures, but your loved one will find comfort in the guidelines, processes, and routines they find throughout their treatment path.

Ask your loved one these questions
- What part of your life would you like to keep the same throughout this process? How can I help you continue with these plans, routines, or activities?
- What new routines can I help you build or honor? Why do these appeal to you right now?

- What helps you feel balance during volatile times? What are some activities that have benefited you in the past when life was stressful or uncertain?
- I know you value following the rules, so can I help you review any information related to upcoming medical appointments, so you understand the norms?

Context

Your loved one with the Context strength is going to need a minute to process their diagnosis. They are reflective and may not kick into action planning and go-forward mode as quickly as you wish. Be patient with their need to uncover background information and details that may help inform their decision-making process. Offer to help them with their research, analyzing, and questioning process.

Take a moment and think about a previous time you heard somebody was diagnosed with cancer or another significant health challenge. More than likely, you probably had questions about the back story. You may have wondered about their symptoms, family history, or the months leading up to their diagnosis. It is common for most of us to want a little context around major life updates, and this desire is magnified for your loved one with Context. Remind yourself that this need for historical grounding will help steady your loved one when they move forward with their cancer treatment and recovery.

Ask your loved one these questions
- What part of your family health history would you like me to help gather? Are there specific family members you'd like me to contact to share your diagnosis?
- What items or memories would you like me to help capture or save? Do you want photographs of your treatment, such as chemotherapy or surgery recovery? Should I record dates certain phases of treatment are completed for you to remember in the future?

- Do you want me to find a place for storage, such as a filing system or box, for the information you'll gather or the items you may receive, such as notes and cards?
- As you are busy receiving information and analyzing your medical decisions, is there any history you'd like me to gather? Do you want more context on the institutions you're considering, the credentials of potential physicians or medical professionals, the type of cancer you have, or the progress made in treatment over the years?

Deliberative

Your loved one with the Deliberative strength is a great decision-maker. Their cancer experience will provide them with plenty of opportunities to use this strength. You have probably observed their pragmatic and thorough decision-making process over the years. Challenge yourself to think of examples and what helped them with those decisions. Did they reach out to experts for insight? Did they spend time alone weighing their options? Did they talk through their thoughts with you, family members, or friends? Provide a few of these specific examples to your loved one to remind them of this strength so they can recreate those past successful processes.

Give them time to think before answering questions. This may be especially important during care team appointments. When you are at these appointments, be prepared to ask probing questions of the providers, take notes, and help your person anticipate the questions they'd like to ask in advance of the session. Rushing them to decisions is probably not helpful, so create time and space for them to arrive there on their own timeline.

Ask your loved one these questions
- What options are you considering? Would you like to pursue a second or third opinion or are you comfortable with your current choices?
- What support can I provide you as you think through your care decisions? Do you want me to listen to your thoughts, share my questions, or do any research for you?

- How can I help you create time in your schedule or a comfortable space for you to do your best thinking?
- I know you value safety and reducing risk, so how can I help you feel better about the options you're considering? Would you like more information, more opinions, or more time to think?
- What risks do you anticipate with your treatment plan? Are there any steps you can take to reduce the risk?

Developer

Your loved one with the Developer strength is a natural teacher, mentor, coach, and supporter. You have probably observed how they help others grow and improve. They will still be driven to do this, even with their cancer diagnosis. If you are concerned about their focus on others, remind yourself that they have always looked for ways to help people develop. Even though it seems counterintuitive, focusing on supporting others will fill them up and be energy giving rather than energy zapping. Be there to support them and recognize this valuable trait of theirs by telling them what you see and appreciate.

Since your person is typically the one helping and supporting others, there could be a possibility that receiving assistance is challenging. You may need to encourage them that accepting help and prioritizing rest is a necessary step toward recovery and getting back to helping others.

Ask your loved one these questions
- What lessons are you being taught by your cancer experience? Do you want to share those with anyone now or down the road?
- Have you noticed anyone on your medical team providing great care? Do you want to recognize them through a card, small gift, or hospital award nomination, like the DAISY Award?[78] The DAISY Award is "a recognition program to thank nurses for the care and kindness they provide and celebrate nurses by collecting nominations from patients and families."

---

78 DAISY Award: https://www.daisyfoundation.org/about-daisy-award.

- How are you supporting people in your life outside of your cancer experience? Are there new opportunities where you'd like to provide guidance based on this new medical experience?
- You are so good at helping and supporting people in their learning and growing journey. If you turned that support inward, what coaching would you give yourself? Is there anything that you'd like to learn that will contribute to your well-being, like meditation, yoga, gardening, or cooking nutritious meals?

Discipline

Your loved one with the strength of Discipline is best served when things are organized and controlled. Their otherwise structured and predictable life may feel wobbly, which can be very hard for them. Show you care by acknowledging that this unplanned health crisis is difficult and stressful, especially for an expert planner.

They will be looking for ways to control the activities and tasks related to cancer. Allow them the time and space to get their arms around the diagnosis, treatment plan, and associated timelines. Your person thrives when they can prepare for what's ahead and accomplish what they need to in a timely manner. They will approach cancer just like they plan projects, vacations, and celebrations. Their approach will be thoughtful, detailed, organized, and near perfect. Let them work their magic to control what they can throughout this process and offer help in creating calmness and structure where you can. For example, if you are more of a night owl and they typically initiate the winding down process in the evenings, give them a thoughtful hand by turning off the TV, dimming the lights, and doing the house closing activities for the night. This is a subtle nod that you see and appreciate their routines and want to help initiate this peaceful serenity too.

Ask your loved one these questions
- What part of your work or personal schedule needs to change and what needs to stay the same? How can I help you adapt plans or keep previously scheduled activities?

- How can I help you feel organized? Are there errands to run, groceries to grab, or communications to be managed that will help you feel in control?
- What new routines can I help you build or honor? For example, if you are focused on getting 10,000 steps a day or 150 minutes of exercise a week, what can I do to help you build that into your daily routine?
- What can I do to help you create an organizing system for new things such as medical receipts, prescriptions, physical therapy exercises, or medical equipment?

Empathy

Your loved one with Empathy talents is emotionally aware and their cancer experience will likely bring out many feelings. They will quickly pick up on how their family, friends, colleagues, neighbors, and doctors are feeling about their diagnosis and treatment outcomes. Processing how other people are feeling is not always a bad thing for a cancer patient. They will experience positive emotions from the heartfelt actions and caring words of others, assuming they have a healthy support system. It can also be validating for them to see and hear others expressing that their condition is serious, and they will help provide needed support. However, if other's reactions become too much for them to hear or witness, encourage them to limit their contact or communications with those people, at least temporarily.

Your loved one is comfortable discussing feelings and emotions. When appropriate, ask them about how they feel. If you are also naturally empathetic, this experience will increase your connection. If you are less empathetic or even struggle to feel and discuss emotions, share that with your loved one. They likely already know this about you, but you may need to ask them to initiate discussions around how cancer is impacting each of you and your relationship.

Ask your loved one these questions
- After medical appointments or cancer-related discussions, ask, "What are you sensing? What does your gut tell you?" Help them stay in tune with their intuition through these prompts.
- Instead of asking, "How are you doing," try asking, "How are you feeling today?" Or ask, "How are you feeling about your appointments

this week?" Aim to be more specific with your questions, which will allow them to be more specific about their feelings, given they have a lot of them.
- How can I help you create a space reflective of your desired mood, such as peaceful, serene, powerful, or bright?
- Who is positively or negatively impacting how you feel? How can I help you spend more or less time with those individuals, accordingly?
- Is there a cancer-related topic I can research or find more data for you? Would you like me to help you brainstorm objective questions before your next appointment?

Focus

Your loved one with the Focus strength is goal-driven and great at avoiding distractions as they zero in on what they want to accomplish. Pay attention to how they frame their cancer diagnosis. Does it feel like they are incorporating it into their life and adjusting their previous goals seamlessly? Does it feel like they are obsessing over it and becoming overly focused on cancer to the exclusion of the rest of their life? Or does it feel like they are ignoring it and moving along with their previous goals as if nothing has happened? Of course, they may exhibit a variety of these attitudes depending on the day and their mindset. As a caregiver, work to engage in conversations around their goals, priorities, distractions, and how they are making adjustments for their diagnosis.

Keep in mind that your person is energized by efficiency. Consider how you can help bring that quality to their cancer experience. For example, can you pick up their prescriptions so they can take a nap instead? While there are aspects of the healthcare system that are out of your control, where can you make a positive impact for your loved one? If you can infuse a little productivity into their time sitting in a waiting room, that could help offset their frustration with the waiting game. Even seemingly small wins of making progress on a goal or recovering a little time back in a waiting room can be a big energy boost for somebody with the Focus strength.

Ask your loved one these questions
- What new goals do you have related to your cancer diagnosis, treatment plan, or overall health and well-being?

- What are your top priorities this week? Is there anything I can help you move forward or do more efficiently?
- Is there anything distracting you from your health-related or personal goals right now? How can I help?
- What would help you see the progress you're making in your cancer experience or the goals you accomplish on the way? Can I help you create something to track that progress?

Futuristic

With Futuristic talents, your loved one's instinct is to look forward. It may feel like they are in denial, downplaying the seriousness of their condition, or diminishing their pain, but looking forward is what gives them energy and strength. Conversations about what they want to do months and years from now may be more beneficial and motivating to them than dwelling on the current state.

Encourage your person to make space to plan and dream. Whether it's reading, writing, daydreaming, or creating, this time will be beneficial to their mood. Engage in conversations about what's ahead and why it excites them. You may not be ready to hear your loved one's view of what's in store as it could include discussions of cancer recurring or planning for disability or death. That can be hard to hear. Do your best to stay open and listen, while also taking care of yourself. Honor what they see and share. Know this is some of the best support you can provide.

Ask your loved one these questions
- What can I do today to help improve your health-related visions and desired outcomes?
- What do you wish existed today that would help you feel better physically or mentally? Their response may provide you with an opening to research helpful options.
- What are your hopes and dreams? Who needs to hear these, and how can I help connect you or create that opportunity? What can you create to keep those dreams visible?
- What do you see next on your treatment path? How can I help you prepare for things you're already anticipating?

Harmony

Your loved one with Harmony talents is naturally calm and steady. They prefer a no-drama approach to life and cancer. Not one to get too high or too low, be prepared for them to handle the news of their diagnosis or treatment with the same calm demeanor. They take a logical, here-and-now approach to processing events and experiences. Do your best to follow their lead in terms of emotions and energy.

Keep in mind that your person is naturally agreeable and looks to experts to help with decision-making. While this collaborative spirit has probably served them well, make sure they aren't going along with recommendations just to avoid conflict. Be prepared to suggest that they may need more information, insight from another provider, or an appointment at a different cancer center. Your loved one is energized by consensus and gaining support for decisions, so you may need to help them work through scenarios of differing medical advice or opinions. While you don't need to have the answers, listening and being by their side as they weigh their options is the best support you can provide.

Ask your loved one these questions
- Are you considering all your treatment options or do you need to seek more opinions? Getting a second or third opinion does not mean that you disagree with the first. You may receive conflicting recommendations, and that is okay. I will support you as you work through your decision.
- What helps you feel balanced, physically and emotionally, right now? How can you incorporate more of those activities or habits into your life, and how can I help?

- I know you value practicality, so can I help you with anything that feels inefficient or is weighing you down?
- Are there any people in your life who are making waves or creating unnecessary friction? What can I do to reduce this tension or how can I best support you through it?
- How can I help you create an ideal space that honors your desire for peace and calm?

Ideation

Your loved one with the Ideation strength is a creative spirit who loves coming up with new ideas, projects, or perspectives. They don't like feeling constrained by the status quo or doing things just because it's the way they have always been done. Pay close attention to their cancer experience and notice what appears to be new and fresh as well as what looks to be stale. Do your best to encourage your person to leverage their creativity and innovative thinking. You may not be the best one for them to ideate with but recommend they connect with another creative friend or group.

Keep in mind that the person you're helping is an outside of the box thinker, so their cancer experience may look a little different from others you have observed or what you imagine someone with cancer will act like. That's not only okay, but ideal to keep them sharp and engaged in their healing.

Ask your loved one these questions
- Where do you do your best thinking and brainstorming? Can I help you create a thinking space at home or somewhere else that appeals to you, like a library or café?
- How can I help bring one of your health-related ideas to life? Are there any steps I can take to move your vision forward?
- What are you curious about related to your cancer or treatment experience? Is there anything you'd like to research or explore further? What can I do to help you organize your ideas related to your health and wellness?
- What is something new or spontaneous you'd like to try, either on your appointment days or days where your energy is best?

Includer

Your loved one with Includer talents thrives on noticing people who are overlooked and bringing everyone into the circle of whatever they are doing. As they go through their cancer experience, you may observe this natural tendency. Whether they are contemplating who to invite along to a doctor's appointment or why a certain demographic has a higher death rate from one type of cancer, their heart is always in the beautiful place of inclusion. Although involving everyone in everything is never possible, honor their positive intent by wanting to include more people, especially those who may be left out. Ask questions to clarify what they desire and try to support their requests when they are aligned with their best health outcomes.

Ask your loved one these questions

- As you learn more about your diagnosis and make care decisions, are there any other experts, cancer survivors, or research articles you would like to consult as you evaluate your options?
- Who would you like to involve in your cancer experience and how should they be included? Are there work colleagues or friends from your faith community you would like me to invite to participate in anything, such as the meal train or rides to radiation?
- Do you feel like anyone is left out of your life right now that you want to spend time with or include in receiving your health updates? What is the best way of contacting this person?
- Are you curious about what somebody is thinking, whether that is a member of your care team, a coworker, or one of your children? Should we brainstorm ways to ask them about their thoughts?

- Is there anyone you prefer to be kept out of your circle of cancer updates and communications? I can help share this preference of yours with anyone who needs to know.

Individualization

Your loved one with Individualization talents is curious about people and likes to learn what makes them tick. Encourage connection as they are going through their cancer experience. They will enjoy meeting members of their care team and others supporting their care. Take note of how they light up a little when they learn new things about their care providers. Make sure to stay engaged in these conversations even if they feel like small talk. They are actually important to your loved one as they will want to feel like they are in great hands as they engage with medical professionals.

Outside of their cancer treatment, you may observe their relationships with friends, family, or colleagues going to a deeper level. This is one of the greatest gifts that came out of my cancer experience, and I think that the strength of Individualization was continuously fed by the time I got to spend with my supporters.

Ask your loved one these questions
- What do you want to know about your current health beyond your cancer diagnosis to perhaps find a more customized treatment plan? How can I help you learn more?
- How do you want people to treat you now that you are a cancer survivor? They may know other cancer survivors who wanted a certain type of support. What is the flavor of support you most need?
- What would you like to know about any of your care team members? What are you curious about their background or experience?
- How can I be of the most support to you? Where do you most want me to spend my time?
- Are there any supporters you're looking forward to getting to know better? How can I best help coordinate more time with them for you?

Input

Your loved one with Input talents will naturally want to consume a lot of information related to their cancer diagnosis. Try to understand they are energized by this process. They may ask for your help with finding books, articles, or websites to help them make medical decisions or research tools to help them through treatment. Depending on your strengths, this may be exciting, fun, boring, or annoying to you. Just keep in mind that the acquisition of information will help your loved one make more informed and confident health-related decisions.

The challenge with the Input strength typically comes with organizing and managing information, whether it's in electronic or physical format. This is an area where you can provide support through advice, encouragement, or action. Be proactive and read about ways to organize medical information, connect with other caregivers on this topic, or ask a nurse navigator or support team member what they've seen work well for other cancer survivors. After appointments, help your loved one review the information they learned, organize any written or electronic materials, and have a solid plan for next steps.

Ask your loved one these questions
- What information do you need today? Can I help you gather any of it—like screenshots, memes, photos—online or by phone?
- What questions would you like to ask your doctor today? I can take notes of their responses and listen for areas to follow up.
- What can I do to help you create a system for all the knowledge you're uncovering? Can I create a physical space at home or buy a small filing box or storage box?

- Are there things you need more information about that I could research and save you time?
- What can I do to help you avoid information overload? Can you delegate or reroute certain people or topics in my direction?

Intellection

Your loved one with Intellection talents is a thinker. Keep in mind that they not only need extra time to think, but they are going to feel better when given that time. Work to help them create routines, structures, and boundaries that allow them time for reflection and time alone to recharge.

You may have experienced times in the past where your loved one was physically in the room, but their mind was far away. It's best not to take this personally, worry that your loved one isn't okay, or assume they don't want to talk to you. People with Intellection tend to be very comfortable with silence, so don't pressure yourself to fill the silence by talking. This is common for people with the strength of Intellection and might increase as they grapple with cancer. Do your best to clarify their needs by asking direct questions so you can assist their thinking process in the most beneficial way for their health. Once you've asked the question, remember you may not receive an answer immediately. In fact, your loved one will probably provide a better answer if you give them a little time.

Ask your loved one these questions
- When and where do you do your best thinking? I want to honor your need for time alone.
- How can I help you ensure your recurring thoughts and questions are captured to bring to the appropriate member of your care team? Do you want me to gather your notes before your upcoming appointments?

- How can you create space in your schedule for this diagnosis and necessary decisions to be made? Are there other commitments that need to be canceled, delayed, or rescheduled to make space?
- Are you open to phone calls and visitors, or would you prefer time alone right now?

Learner

Your loved one with Learner talents is a student for life. This will help them tremendously as they are thrust into the world of cancer. The main support you can provide is asking them questions to spark their curiosity. Offer to support them in the learning process whether that is taking on some of the online research, reaching out to cancer-related organizations, or compiling any of their learnings. The sheer volume of information can be overwhelming. If you find your loved one appears to want to learn everything, help them prioritize what's most important to explore, what can be saved for later, and what may be interesting but is irrelevant. They may push back, but boundaries for learning are important, especially given their likely reduced energy levels.

Many people with the Learner strength enjoy cutting-edge knowledge or technology along with variety. Engage them in conversations about the science and medical aspects of their treatment plan. Be prepared for them to get bored with too much repetition, especially if their plan includes a long stretch of the same activity, such as 30 days of radiation.

Ask your loved one these questions
- Is any part of your treatment plan or process feeling boring or mundane? How can we freshen things up, so it feels new?
- What can I do to help you create a system for all the knowledge you're uncovering? Can I create a physical space at home or buy a small filing box or storage box?
- Are there products, processes, or resources you need more information about that I could research and save you time?

- What are you curious about related to cancer, health, or survivorship and what would be the best way for you to learn about it? How can I help?
- What is most important to learn more about right now? What could wait for later?
- How can I help you apply what you've learned? Can I help you develop questions for your care team from what you've learned to see how it relates to your treatment?

Maximizer

Your loved one with Maximizer talents is focused on improving, raising the bar, and moving toward quality and excellence. They will not lose that edge during their cancer experience, but you may need to help them adjust their high expectations of themselves and others. As they consider their care team and treatment plan options, pay attention to their level of satisfaction by making note of their facial expressions and nonverbal reactions, or directly asking them how good they feel about their team and the plan. People with the Maximizer strength can get frustrated with average performance, mediocrity, and the status quo. If you sense they are less than satisfied with their experience, it may be time to regroup and explore a second or third opinion or express these concerns with the care team. If they feel confident in their care center, medical providers, and treatment plan, that is a great sign! Validate that they have made great selections about their healthcare options.

Ask your loved one these questions
- How can I help make your cancer experience better? Is there something that can be improved with your appointment processes, organizing information, or health-related communications with friends and family?
- What was the best part of your recent visit? What, if anything, could your care team be doing to make your patient experience better?
- Where do you feel like you need to let go of a few responsibilities to conserve energy? How can I or others help take over those tasks or are they things that can be dropped for the time being?

- Is there an area of your life where you'd like to focus on making improvements? For example, do you want to start walking outside more often or cooking one meal a week as a family?

Positivity

Your loved one with Positivity talents is energetic and optimistic, and you may often see them as happy and fun to be around. Those are not necessarily the first descriptions that come to mind when people think about a cancer patient. As positive as your person can be, you may also see them wrestling with their disease. Try to make space for both experiences while supporting their desire to take a glass-half-full approach. They will want to engage with people and live life to the fullest while also being realistic about their treatment. Have conversations with them about how you can best help to support their desire to take a hopeful approach.

People with the Positivity strength are often sensitive to the moods of others, so do your part to reduce potential negative vibes. A critical component of being a caregiver is taking care of yourself as well. Supporting a loved one through a cancer experience can be mentally and emotionally draining. Do your best to take care of your own well-being so that you aren't bogged down by fatigue, stress, sadness, or fear.

Ask your loved one these questions
- What are the three things you're grateful for today? What were your wins for the week?
- Is there anything fun you want to do during this next phase of your treatment?
- How does a celebration for a cancer win or milestone sound to you? What would a perfect celebration look like to you?
- Is there any negativity surrounding you that I can help diffuse or deflect? Please let me know how to help create the most positive experience possible for you.

Relator

Your loved one with Relator talents will likely approach their cancer diagnosis the same way they have approached other challenges and life adversities, with their closest friends and family by their side. Check in with them frequently and allow time for conversations to extend deeper, beyond the basics of how the day was and how they are feeling. They cherish quality time with people they love. Make time for these moments and conversations. Remind them how deeply you care for them and will support them in whatever way feels best.

Your person is genuine and authentic and will approach cancer with that style as well. Avoid clichés and generalizations when speaking about their disease and treatment plan. They will set the tone for how they prefer to discuss their health but be prepared for it to be real and vulnerable. Listening carefully and asking good questions is the best support you can provide your loved one with the Relator strength. Knowing they are truly being heard and not seen as just another cancer patient will be very important along the way.

Ask your loved one these questions
- Who would you like to spend the most time with as you go through your treatment process? Do you want me to help coordinate this time together?
- What part of your cancer experience would you like to keep private? Is there anything you share with me that you do not want repeated to anyone else or kept within your small circle?

- Have you met a care provider or cancer survivor that you'd like to get to know better? What is a good next step to build that relationship further, and how can I help support you?
- I know you value authenticity, so what would make your cancer experience feel more genuine, real, and authentic? Is there anything you're hearing or feeling from supporters that doesn't resonate with you?

Responsibility

Your loved one with Responsibility talents still needs to honor their commitments and be true to their word. They are energized by knowing that others see them as trustworthy, reliable, and dependable. That confidence from others fuels them to complete their obligations. While they may not be able to do everything they were doing prior to their diagnosis, allow them the freedom to decide what tasks they'll let go of or modify. Asking for help is difficult for many people, but it's especially difficult for those with this strength. Be patient.

Instead of making assumptions about where they need your help, either give them a few choices or let them guide you to what they need. Delegating, prioritizing, and setting boundaries will be critical skillsets for your person during this cancer experience. Watch for opportunities to support them without trying to strip them of their commitments.

Your person will likely have no problem following the recommendations of their care team. If they commit to something during an appointment, such as exercising 150 minutes per week, they will do it. You can be inspired by their commitment. Consider ways to recognize their dedication and highlight their strength.

Ask your loved one these questions
- What commitments are overwhelming you right now? Can you remove, revise, or revisit these commitments?
- What can I take off your plate? Are there a few things you can delegate my way?
- What boundaries can I help you honor? Would you like me to check in with you to make sure you are sticking to these limits?

- What cancer or medical related actions have you taken this week? Can we take a moment to celebrate your commitment to your health?
- Are you feeling smothered or micromanaged by people who mean well? I know you value having freedom to do things independently, so how can we respectfully let them know to give you space?

Restorative

Your loved one with Restorative talents is a natural problem solver. They know that life comes with problems, issues, and challenges. They aren't rattled by problems; in fact, solving them fuels your loved one. Keep this in mind as they are going through their cancer experience. Life will continue, and they may face challenges in addition to managing their cancer diagnosis. While you might be tempted to jump in and save the day, ask if they'd like your help first. Fixing things and solving everyday problems, while draining for some, is energizing to someone with this strength. Check in to see if they want your help, if they want to handle it themselves, or if they'd enjoy taking a collaborative approach and fixing it together.

Ask your loved one these questions
- What feels off to you in your life? For example, are you missing your exercise classes or your time spent gardening? How can I help you restore what is feeling off?
- Is there anything broken that you'd like to see fixed? I can handle a home repair project, an IT challenge, or a car checkup if that would help you feel better.
- Is there any part of you that feels physically painful? Are you having challenges due to side effects of treatment or medication? Is this something that could be improved with a complementary therapy, like massage, acupuncture, physical therapy, or stretching?

Self-Assurance

Your loved one with Self-Assurance talents is typically calm and controlled. Do not be surprised if they approach their cancer diagnosis the same way—it's their strength! They do well with challenges, are willing to take risks, make difficult decisions, and feel confident being in the driver's seat of their own life. Be by their side as they move through their cancer experience and be comfortable with the fact that they might not need a lot of help from you and others. That's a sign that their Self-Assurance strength is helping internally guide them through this challenge—and that's a great thing.

Ask your loved one these questions
- As you consider your treatment plan options, what's your gut telling you? What you feel right now might not be your final decision, but I'd love to know what you are feeling today.
- You are usually certain in your decisions. Is there anything you're uncertain about? Is there anything you're unsure about related to your new schedule, potential side effects, or next steps? What would help you feel more confident about these things?
- What information do you need to make one of your health-related decisions? Do you want me to help research anything or connect you with an expert?
- I'm so impressed with how calm you are as you make care decisions. What's helped you be that way over the years? What happens within you or around you when you are making your best decisions?

Significance

Your loved one with Significance talents values being seen and heard. One of the best things you can do is to carefully watch and listen to how they're navigating their cancer experience. Share what you see and what you find interesting, fascinating, and inspiring. They will appreciate your close attention to their experiences, as they won't want to be lumped in with other cancer patients you've known.

Supporters may want to shower your loved one with gifts, meals, and attention. While they typically don't shy away from an audience, get their approval in advance in case they have opinions about the details. For example, people may offer to provide weekly meals for your family, but your loved one may prefer they put that money toward a local Relay for Life team or support a local youth with cancer. Your loved one is an incredible dreamer and difference-maker, so keep their thoughts at the forefront throughout the process. You will probably be amazed at the outcomes.

Additionally, people with this strength are driven to make an impact and leave a legacy. Cancer often brings people a little closer to considering their mortality and examining their life's purpose. Your loved one likely had a bit more clarity, or at least consideration, around these big life topics prior to their diagnosis. Keep in mind that impact and difference making has always been important to them and cancer may amplify that desire.

Ask your loved one these questions
- What's most important to you now? How can I help you make time for those people or activities?

- How can we help you appreciate and celebrate cancer milestones, such as completing a cycle of chemotherapy, finishing radiation, or a successful surgery?
- Are there any places or audiences where you'd like to be seen as a cancer survivor? For example, do you want us to create a relay team for the local cancer organization 5K? Do you want to speak at a cancer support group? How can I help?
- What goals or accomplishments do you want to focus on during this cancer experience? Are there personal or work-related goals you still want to achieve? Are there new health-related goals that I can support or provide accountability?
- What part of your cancer experience or daily life would you like to do independently? I know you value freedom and space, so let me help you achieve that where it makes sense.
- Who are you comfortable seeing during the most challenging parts of this medical process? What's your preferred way of connection from your supporters? Do you want them to go for coffee or a walk, text or call, or visit in person?

Strategic

Your loved one with Strategic talents is naturally a big picture thinker. They can take a project, challenge, or initiative and quickly see all the different options, pathways, and scenarios from beginning to end. Do not be surprised if they approach their cancer diagnosis as a project like any other. They will spend more time thinking and talking about the larger phases of their treatment than the specific details of one day or one event.

While you may worry they are in denial, they are more likely facing cancer tactically and creatively, the way they face other parts of their life. Feel free to ask questions about how they are making their decisions but also trust them to be taking all the moving parts into consideration.

Ask your loved one these questions
- When you think about the big picture of this cancer diagnosis, where do you think you will need support? Do you think you will need help at work, with household responsibilities, community commitments, or with your obligations to your loved ones?
- I know you can feel depleted when faced with the minutiae of larger projects or efforts. Are there any small details or tasks of your cancer care that I can do for you?
- Is there anything that your supporters are concerned about that you've already moved past? For example, people may be worried about you missing out on a fun event or dealing with losing your hair and your changing appearance. I can let them know to let go of these concerns since your thoughts move quickly and you have already moved past those challenges.

- When you zoom out of this current health challenge, what do you see? I'd love to hear your thoughts from that bird's-eye view if you're open to sharing.

Woo

Your loved one with Woo talents is no doubt a known force in your family, friend circle, neighborhood, and community. People with this strength may move through their cancer experience in the same way they always have, by making new friends along the way. Or they may prefer to turn toward their inner circle of closer connections. Whatever people-approach they prefer, honor it. Their appetite for chatting, meeting new people, and creating or participating in fun activities may ebb and flow through their cancer experience. Continue to check in with them on their people-related needs, and support their preferences for connection or privacy, new connections or established friendships, and fun activities or calm rest.

Your person is energized by being around other people. If you sense they are overexerting themselves to socialize or putting their immunity at risk by being in large groups, check in with them on their motivation. Are they intentionally prioritizing being with people because it fuels them or because it's what they've always done? While you don't need to be the Fun Police, you can check in on how they are balancing socializing and rest.

Ask your loved one these questions
- What are three concerns you have related to your cancer diagnosis, and who do you know who may be able to help?
- Which connections would you like to hear the news of your diagnosis, and how would you like that information shared?
- Is there anyone you know who you do not want to hear about your diagnosis or treatment updates?

- Is there anyone new outside your network you'd like to meet? What's the best way for you to meet them, and how can I help make it happen?
- Would you like fun incorporated into your treatment plan or your life outside the cancer center? What feels appropriate to you on that front, and what feels out of bounds—even on your fun-o-meter?

Resources for Surviving Cancer with Your Strengths

A full list of books, references, and other useful material is available at https://followyourstrengths.com/book.

Introduction

National Cancer Institute website: https://www.cancer.gov

American Cancer Society: https://www.cancer.org

Jeremy Pietrocini and Benjamin Erikson-Farr, Gallup Clifton Strengths (June 23, 2015) *Learn, Love, Live: The Journey of Strengths.* Available at: https://www.gallup.com/cliftonstrengths/en/251093/learn-love-live-journey-strengths.aspx

Stuart Scott, V Foundation (2014) "When You Die, It Does Not Mean That You Lose to Cancer." Available at: https://www.v.org/story/when-you-die-it-does-not-mean-that-you-lose-to-cancer-stuart-scott/

Part One: Strengths, Mindset, and Cancer

For more about Dr. Donald Clifton's revolutionary approach of helping to identify the good in people: Gallup CliftonStrengths, *Learn About the History of CliftonStrengths.* Available at: https://www.gallup.com/cliftonstrengths/en/253754/history-cliftonstrengths.aspx

For more on Jim Clifton, Dr. Donald Clifton's son and former CEO of Gallup, see Gallup (2007) *StrengthsFinder 2.0,* "Discover Your CliftonStrengths." Gallup Press https://www.followyourstrengths.com/book

For more about the impact on people's lives when they have the opportunity to use their strengths see Gallup CliftonStrengths, *Learn About the Science and Validity of CliftonStrengths*. Available at: https://www.gallup.com/cliftonstrengths/en/253790/science-of-cliftonstrengths.aspx

Turner, Kelly A. (2015) *Radical Hope: 10 Key Healing Factors from Exceptional Survivors of Cancer & Other Diseases*. Reprint. HarperOne.

Turner, Kelly A. (2014) *Radical Remission: Surviving Cancer Against All Odds*. HarperOne.

For books by Tom Rath such as *How Full Is Your Bucket?*, *StrengthsFinder 2.0*, *Strengths Based Leadership*, *Are You Fully Charged?* and *Wellbeing: The Five Essential Elements*, visit https://www.followyourstrengths.com/book

Gallup's Values cards: https://www.followyourstrengths.com/book

Clifton, D. O. and Nelson, P. (1992) *Soar with Your Strengths: A Simple yet Revolutionary Philosophy of Business and Management*. 6th edition. Delacorte Press.

Part Two: 34 Strengths, Cancer Connections, Considerations, and Cautions

For more about ACS CAN, the American Cancer Society Cancer Action Network: https://www.fightcancer.org/about

CaringBridge: https://www.caringbridge.org/

ACS CARES™, American Cancer Society: https://www.cancer.org/support-programs-and-services/acs-cares.html

Breast Cancer Advocacy, National Breast Cancer Coalition: https://www.stopbreastcancer.org/

Mukherjee, Siddhartha (2010) *The Emperor of All Maladies: A Biography of Cancer*. Scribner.

DIEP Flap Breast Reconstruction for Natural Breasts: https://prma-enhance.com/breast-reconstruction/diep-flap

NCI Dictionary of Cancer Terms: https://www.cancer.gov/publications/dictionaries/cancer-terms

Izzy Wheels, Wheelchair Wheel Covers: https://www.izzywheels.com/

Kate Bowler: https://katebowler.com

Look Good Feel Better: https://lookgoodfeelbetter.org/

NCI-Designated Cancer Centers: https://www.cancer.gov/research/infrastructure/cancer-centers

Pink Pockets™, Post Mastectomy Drain Holders: www.pink-pockets.com

Everest, Laura, *Rebuilt to Last: Choose to Flourish*, Notion Press 2021

Can Do Cancer, Iowa: https://candocancer.org/

American Cancer Society Road to Recovery® program, American Cancer Society https://www.cancer.org/support-programs-and-services/road-to-recovery.html

American Cancer Society Cancer Action Network: https://www.fightcancer.org/what-we-do/access-biomarker-testing

Thich Nhat Hanh, Plum Village: https://plumvillage.org/about/thich-nhat-hanh

Kristin Neff, Self-Compassion: https://self-compassion.org

Cancer Action Network (ACS CAN), American Cancer Society: https://www.cancer.org/involved/volunteer/acs-can.html

Part Three: Caregiver Considerations

For more about caregiver resources from the American Cancer Society: https://www.cancer.org/cancer/caregivers.html

For more about caregiver resources from the National Cancer Institute: https://www.cancer.gov/about-cancer/coping/caregiver-support.html

For more about caregiver resources from Cancer*Care*:
https://www.cancercare.org/tagged/caregiving.html

Note: All links in this book were accessed on November 1, 2025 unless otherwise noted.

Acknowledgments

Thank you so much to the team who brought this book to life in full color. Jen Louden, I'm so glad I hired you as my book coach when I saw Shannon Watts's Instagram story about you. Given that Activator is your top strength, but 32 of 34 for me, your energy was the perfect match to help me move this project forward. You pushed me to add examples and stories from other cancer survivors, and it was just what the book needed. The rest of the team came from your recommendations and network... you were essentially the team captain, thank you! Ruth Bullivant, thank you for the energy you put into editing and creating the index. Your idea to add headings to the considerations sections was brilliant and made the book better for the reader. Your Input and Deliberative strengths were evident in the careful attention you gave to every single resource, citation, and reference. Carra Simpson, you had your work cut out for you to manage the timeline and keep me on track. I appreciate the empathy you brought to our conversations in the final weeks when I struggled with overwhelm, doubt, and not feeling ready to let the book go. I'm thankful for your thoroughness and attention to detail every step of the way. Eva van Emden, thank you for your proofreading expertise and multiple passes through the manuscript. Words matter. I loved when you caught words or phrases that had nuanced meanings. Carra and I had fun discussions around many of those and especially enjoyed "doughnut" versus "donut." Jazmin Welch, I couldn't love the cover more. Thank you for your patience as we worked through all the options. Your Positivity strength was evident throughout our time working together. Alex Hennig, the book interior turned out so great thanks to you. I appreciated your chill vibe and easygoing nature as timelines shifted. I didn't even need to see Adaptability in your strengths profile to know you had it!

To the cancer survivors who shared your stories with me—thank you for taking the time to reflect on your cancer experiences and think about how your strengths impacted some of your decisions, actions, struggles, and successes. I know it was a tough ask to either take you back to when you were going through cancer or examine how you're currently feeling navigating cancer. So I appreciate you going there with me and candidly sharing your uniqueness and resilience on these pages. Generous cancer survivors who shared their stories include Chris Baker, Erica Bergfeld-Reed, Dr. Giulia Bonaminio, Christine Carpenter, Diane Chandler, Sarah Corkery, Barb Curran, Gina D'Errico Brennan, Melanie Dean, Deb Eisloeffel, Ashley Flynn, Mary Sue Ingraham, Sharon Juon, Autumn Kline, Holly LaVallie, Donna Lewondowski, Jennifer McLamb, Donna O'Brien, Josie Orrick, Angie Owen, Jennifer Pihlaja, Dr. Melissa Reade, Michelle Richardson, Kathy Simon, Carrie Skowronski, Dave Smith, Andrea Spudich, Kristin Teig Torres, Tara Tvedt, Holly Van Fleet, Traci Wagner, Catherine Watson, and Amy Wienands. Also thank you to those who shared how their strengths helped them through severe physical injuries, including Charlotte Blair, Laura Everest, and Richelle Leaming. Also thank you to the countless survivors not named specifically in the book whose stories I heard or read about over the years. Your experiences helped shape my thoughts, insights, and questions.

To the Gallup team—wow. To state the obvious, this book wouldn't exist without your IP and the groundbreaking work of Dr. Don Clifton. For you to grant me an official Gallup Content License to help other cancer survivors is a real gift. Jon Clifton and Jim Clifton, thank you for your incredible support of the book and for championing its reach in the world. Seth Schuchman, you breathed life into my book idea and early writings during our first meeting in 2018. Both you and Jessica Kennedy-Matthews continued your positive encouragement to "Keep going!" and "Write the book!" when I would see you at the annual Gallup at Work Summit through the years. Thank you for believing in the idea, sharing advice, and taking time to guide me through the process. Scott

Wright, thank you for your support with content licensing and your initiative in helping with the flow and readability of the strengths content. Jim Asplund, thank you for your positive feedback about the book from the perspective of a cancer survivor and one of Gallup's top strengths experts. It meant so much and gave me a boost in momentum during the months of critical review and editing that followed. Jim Collison, you have been such a great friend and cheerleader for me over the years. You are the face and friend to the Global Strengths Community, and the amount of time and energy you've put into the podcasting and social media channels has been incredible. Even though I was pretty nervous, I absolutely loved being your podcast guest on *Called to Coach* in 2018 and 2022. Your Woo and Communication strengths helped make the experience a breeze . . . and of course, fun! To you and Adam Hickman, thank you for supporting me in the first Eastern Iowa Meetup and bringing your generous spirit to the room virtually when over 20 people gathered just in the name of . . . strengths. JerLene Mosley, it's been "groovy" to count you as a strengths advisor. I love teachers, and I love that you devoted your career to strengths in schools. Thank you for always making time for a call when I had questions or wanted to introduce you to other rock star educators. Maika Leibbrandt, you poured so much of yourself into making strengths coaches around the world better. Thank you for helping make this book better too. You have such a cool energy about you, and it's been fun to watch you grow on your career, motherhood, and entrepreneur journeys. Paul Allen, thank you for the inspiration and passion you poured into the certified coaching community. Hearing you read *Let the Rabbits Run* from the stage at the 2016 Strengths Summit and your tributes to Dr. Don Clifton over the years have helped fuel my quieter, internal knowing that this work is so important. Tom Rath, thank you for your encouraging words to write this book and for all the positive contributions you've made in the world around strengths, leadership, and well-being.

To my Gallup Strengths teachers, Heather Wright and Curt Liesveld—it's interesting for me to think back to our time together in Omaha in 2014. The week-long certification program with you two as facilitators changed my life forever. I went into it with sort of a gut instinct that this was going to be a good thing for me and my career. But I had no idea that what you taught me would actually *become* my career. I don't know that a combination of any two other teachers would have led me to go all in on strengths in my business. You were magic together. Heather, thank you for coaching me over the years, for meeting me after chemo in Iowa City, and for always making time to catch up in Omaha during the summer. And Curt, I obviously wish I could have known you longer before your passing but am grateful we can all still learn from your teachings through your writings and the original *Theme Thursday* podcasts. You were studying and writing about the concept of light before your passing. Thank you for being a light for me and thousands of other Gallup-Certified Strengths Coaches and practitioners around the world.

To the Gallup-Certified Strengths Coaches around the world—you'd be hard pressed to find a more generous, passionate, supportive group of individuals in another field or industry. After Jim Collison invited me to share on the Coaches Community Call, I posted in the private Facebook group that I was looking for people to help review the strengths chapters. Your response blew me away! Some of you I've known for years and consider friends and colleagues. Others of you I've never met and live in different countries around the world. Nearly 50 of you reviewed the strengths chapters in the book, including Rasha Alajouz, Helen Arthur, Chris Baker, Ken Barr Jr., Charlotte Blair, Gina D'Errico Brennan, Ali Carson, Xander Cladder, Heidi Convery-Liscum, Martin Daubney, Deb Eisloeffel, Laura Everest, Rodrigo Ferreira, Jo Fitzgerald, Donna Gardner, Kathie Gautille, Beverly Griffeth-Bryant, Jeanne Hamra, Barb Hannon, Florence Hardy, Susan Hoover, Mary Sue Ingraham, Michaela Jacobs, Gail Early Jokerst, Katie Kloosterman, Maika Leibbrandt, Donna Lewandowski, Naomi Lippin, Marina Mamshina, Jane McCarthy, Sheri Miter, JerLene Mosley, Siobhan O'Riordan, TyAnn Osborn, Kristen O'Shea, Cheryl Pace, Tracy Phillips, Jennifer Pihlaja, Michelle Richardson, Brea Roper, Nicole Seichter, Carrie Skowronski, Andrea Spudich, Marla Turner, Kat Van Dusen, Catherine Watson, and Dr. Carol

Acknowledgments

Wheeler. I am so grateful to you all for your generosity and abundance mindset while spending time reviewing the strengths chapters.

To the team at Follow Your Strengths—thanks to everyone who has helped this business grow and evolve the last 10+ years. Cally Reed, you were the best intern in the history of interns. You truly grasped the strengths philosophy, and your creativity around work was so inspiring to me during those early years. After you graduated and were in between jobs and I was in a lull of writing this book, it was great to have you and your Strategic Thinking strengths back to gather research and creative ideas. Nikki Allen, one of my favorite memories of the business was having you join me for workshops. Your Woo energy is so fun and contagious, and your Achiever and Competition strengths helped me know you would manage a room or a project in the best way possible. You're amazing, Nik. Megan Droste, they say to look for people with complementary strengths to help you at work. You and I are so similar with our Top 10, but that Discipline strength of yours is exactly what I've needed to get on track and move things forward. Thank you for your support with so many projects along the way to getting this book out into the world. Thank you to the brilliant, creative minds who have helped with our marketing over the years—Sarah Pauls, Gus Pladsen, Hailee Gillett, and Taylor Henry. Thank you to the incredible team at Coefficient Solutions for your support in preparing materials for workshops and speaking events. In particular, thank you so much to Kelly Etter and Veronica Martinez-Goodman. Our business wouldn't be where it is today without the complementary strengths partnership we've had for all these years. The two of you, and your Responsibility strengths, are amazing.

To my business mentors and coaches—Charlotte Blair, Lisa Cummings, Sam Deines, Amy Dutton, Jess Ekstrom, Dr. Christi Hegstad, Maggie Jackson, Lori Johnson, Gale Mote, Dr. Celina Peerman, Erin Peterson, Kendra Richman, Dr. Kristine Sickels, Krischelle Tennessen, and our Lean In Circle. Thanks to each of you whether you gave me guidance, advice, encouragement, or accountability. Most importantly, thank you for believing in me and this book.

To cancer organizations, advocacy groups, and supporters—Sarah Corkery, thank you for being my cancer mentor. You took a call from a stranger in the thick of your radiation treatment during your own cancer journey. It still blows me away that you spent 45 minutes answering all my questions from your room at the American Cancer Society Hope Lodge in Iowa City. Your advice and recommendations on how to prepare for chemo and surgery gave me an edge that almost felt like cheating. Thanks to your Woo strength, you even found me a new friend to face chemo treatments with. Meeting Laurel Hibbard and the three of us staying in touch was one of the highlights of having cancer. Sarah, your honesty was a gift as I navigated through so much information in those early months. Your Communication strength is always on point . . . even when you delivered the tough facts about a terrible disease. I love how we can still laugh about you blatantly dropping facts about recurrence over lunch at Noodles & Company with me when I was bald, tired, and clueless! You are a gem, and thank you for guiding me through cancer and becoming a great friend along the way.

Beyond Pink TEAM amazing women and National Breast Cancer Coalition advocates—you have supported, educated, and inspired me since the early months of my diagnosis. Your work matters and you are all difference makers. Dee Hughes and Gabbi DeWitt, thank you for the love you put into the support group meetings and for letting me use your great book library. I still remember walking in bald, exhausted, and scared for my first meeting and encountering your welcoming and caring hearts. It was a pivotal moment for me during the tough final stretch of my treatment. Christine Carpenter, Sarah Corkery, Beth Drelich, Lori Seawel, Kristin Teig Torres, and Kent McCausland—I'll never forget "walking the halls of Congress" with each of you. Christine, thank you for being our fearless leader, teaching me so much about advocacy, and continuously sharing your important reminder about legislators—"They work for us."

American Cancer Society of Iowa and American Cancer Society Cancer Action Network team Iowa—thanks to each of you for your service as board members and advocates. I've learned so much from you and am excited about the future impact we can help create and support together. A special thank you to Margaret McCaffery for inviting Kent and me to serve on the board. I've loved meeting with our legislators in D.C. with you for ACS CAN. The time and energy you both gave in raising over $2 million to support cancer efforts in Iowa and beyond is so admirable. We are forever grateful for the love and support from your family when I was sick and when we lost Mac.

To the incredible team at UIHC—thank you for showing up to work like you had only one thing in mind each day—your patients. The calm, kind, and respectful energy in the Holden Comprehensive Cancer Center starts with the staff—oncologists, surgeons, schedulers, infusion nurses, lab technicians, researchers, psychologists, pharmacists, and more. I'd specifically like to thank my incredible oncologist, Dr. Sneha Phadke. You gave our family hope with your steady reassurance, always backed by data and research. Your strengths shone so clearly to me, and I'm thankful for your inquisitive and truthful nature with your Learner and Relator strengths. Dr. Sonia Sugg, your presence and brilliance the first time we met solidified our decision to travel to Iowa City for treatment. Your Input, Achiever, and Strategic strengths were so reassuring with each important decision you helped us make along the treatment path. Thank you to Dr. Thomas Lawrence, Dr. Nicole Nisly, Dr. Scott Temple, and Dr. Kathryn Huber-Keener for guiding me through my care for surgery, OBGYN, nutrition, mindset, and survivorship. Also thank you to the care team professionals who have helped me since my diagnosis, specifically Dr. Julia Buchkina, Dr. Marilyn Hines, Dr. Suzanne Bartlett Hackenmiller, Dr. Lauren Whipple, Jenna Berendzen, DNP, and Maryjane Cose, ARNP.

To my amazing friends—this section pains me to not list names. Please write your own name in your favorite color, large font, and all caps because you got me through cancer! A big hug to the Iowa Falls friends of my parents who showed up strong for them as they were filled with worry when I was initially diagnosed. For the Iowa Falls Cadets I grew up with, graduated with (go 1996!), and have continued our friendships—well, "thank you" doesn't come close to cutting it. You called, you texted, you prayed, you sent cards, you cooked, and most importantly . . . you showed up. I will never forget you. To my college and Kansas City friends—I wasn't sure I'd ever make one friend to rival those I made growing up in Iowa Falls. You all outdid yourselves, and I'm lucky to have you in my life. Thank you for the calls, texts, gift cards, and support. KC Crime Family forever. To our Waterloo friends—dang. Your love changed my life. I will always see the good in people more easily because of how good you were to the four of us when I got sick.

To all of these amazing friends—from Iowa Falls to Kansas City to Waterloo—can you even believe everything you did? You sat with us before the diagnosis was even official. You joined me for lunch and wig shopping before my first chemo. You came with me to KJ's for the Farewell to Hair party. You drove me to chemo. You made purple #STRENGTH T-shirts, texted purple hearts, and somehow organized 20 dudes to wear purple polos for Millennium Cup. You took my love of purple and helped me feel truly seen through all the generic pink ribbons. You took me on walks, brought me smoothies, and took the boys to the lake for fun getaways. You walked with me in the Beyond Pink TEAM Pink Ribbon Run. You helped create the most amazing donut wall and waffle bar when we celebrated after the race. You hosted dinners for me before my double mastectomy where we debated implant sizes and enjoyed adorable cupcakes perfectly themed for the occasion. You sent gifts of absolutely everything from scarfs and hats to cozy blankets and clothes to beautiful flowers, bracelets, bags, and books. Your generosity knew no end. Then you blew me away with one of the best surprises of my life—beautiful white Christmas lights hanging on our tall house. You called, texted, prayed, cooked, and again . . . showed up. There is so much good in this world. There is so much beauty in this world. There is so much love in this world. And I am so lucky to have some of that good, beauty, and love in my small little world.

To the Core Four: Dad, Mom, and Bear—I wish we didn't have to go through cancer together, but we definitely went through it together. I knew you had my back the day I was diagnosed, and you were with me every step of the way. Big thanks to the love and support from our entire family—Mac, Linda, Bill, Ryan, Amy, Michael, Molly, Jenna, Brian, Henry, Charlotte, and loving aunts, uncles, and cousins.

To Kenny and the Boys: Whew. Can you believe this book is actually real? Thank you for never questioning the time I put into these pages—even when it meant me taking off for a writing retreat, spending a few days out of town, or all the late nights in my office coming home to sleep about when you were waking up. The amount of love I have for you is what made cancer feel so scary and living feel so special. I love you so much.

Index

A

ACS CAN 74, 112, 255, 336, 337
Advance Care Planning 140
advocacy 44, 73, 74, 75, 84, 93, 103,
    112, 120, 123, 204, 209, 235, 240,
    254, 255
  American Cancer Society 112
  National Breast Cancer Coalition
    112, 336
American Cancer Society 1, 2, 57, 74,
    75, 240, 255, 272, 335, 337
  ACS CARES 91, 336
  Cancer Action Network 240, 336,
    337
  Road to Recovery® 240, 337
American Psychological Association 18
Angelou, Maya, Dr. 251
anxiety 4, 5, 22, 65, 91, 110, 118, 163,
    164, 194
Asplund, J. 31

B

bell, ring the 1, 134, 224, 253, 276, 290
Beyond Pink TEAM 68, 74
biomarker testing 240
Blair, Charlotte 82
Block, Keith, Dr. 22
Bonaminio, Giulia, Dr. 249
Bowler, Kate, Dr. 197, 202, 269, 337
Breast Cancer Awareness 221, 259

C

Calhoun, Lawrence, Dr. 21
Can Do Cancer, Iowa 337

caregiver resources 272
CaringBridge 89, 229, 253, 336
Clifton, Donald, Dr. 13, 15, 16, 18, 28,
    31, 335, 336
Clifton, Jim 15, 18, 335
Collison, Jim 266
Cooling Caps 57
Couric, Katie 61
Crippes, C. 74

D

DAISY Award 299
Dawson, Jessica 33
delegate 43, 51, 192, 216, 234, 246,
    253, 315, 325
Deweese, Cathy 15
DIEP Flap Breast Reconstruction 121,
    206, 215, 337
domain
  Executing 42, 239
  Influencing 264
  Relationship Building 54
  Strategic Thinking 61
Dweck, Carol, Dr. 19, 20

E

Erikson-Farr, Benjamin 11, 335
Everest, Laura 337
Executing domain. *See* Gallup: domain:
    Executing

F

Five Clues to Talent 31
Four E's 31
FranklinCovey 155

G

Gallup
    CliftonStrengths 3, 15, 16, 31, 32, 34, 40, 48, 69, 81, 104, 138, 228, 246, 335, 336
        StrengthsFinder 10, 16, 18, 28, 31, 335, 336
    CliftonStrengths assessment 16, 18, 24, 30, 31, 274
    domain
        Executing 42, 239
        Influencing 264
        Relationship Building 54
        Strategic Thinking 61
    History of CliftonStrengths 16
    Talent Themes 16, 48, 104, 138, 200, 228, 246
    Theme Dynamics 31
    Theme Thursday podcast 104, 189, 200, 228, 246
    Values cards 76
Google 8, 9, 23, 194

H

hair
    damage 135
    Farewell to Hair party 68
    Look Good Feel Better 204
    loss 56, 57, 175, 206, 239, 331

I

Influencing domain. *See* Gallup: domain: Influencing
Ingraham, Mary Sue 27, 102, 104, 190
Izzy Wheels 175, 337

J

Jardin, Xeni 9

K

Kotb, Hoda 218, 220, 221

L

Lasker, Mary 267, 268
    Lasker Foundation 267, 268
LaVallie, Holly 24, 259
legacy 251, 252, 256, 329, 330
Leibbrandt, Maika 81
Liesveld, Curt vii, 11, 48, 69, 138, 189, 228
Look Good Feel Better 204, 337

M

Mayo Clinic 55, 259
mentor 77, 91, 97, 134, 140, 193, 208, 235, 254, 267, 299
mindset 2, 11, 19, 20, 22, 23, 29, 54, 57, 69, 83, 96, 107, 111, 116, 168, 186, 205, 208, 212, 224, 227, 239, 241, 245, 284, 305
Mukherjee, Siddhartha 120, 267

N

nails, damage 135
National Breast Cancer Coalition 73, 74, 193
National Cancer Institute 1, 2, 21, 35, 120, 211, 272, 335, 337
NCI-Designated Cancer Centers 211
NCI Dictionary of Cancer Terms 170, 245, 337
NED. *See* No Evidence of Disease
Neff, Kristin, Dr. 242, 337
No Evidence of Disease 266, 275, 288
nutrition 174, 205, 207, 208, 293

O

Oncology
    dietitian 204
    psychologist 90, 91, 204

P

Pathologic Complete Response. *See* pCR
pCR 121, 170, 171

Phadke, Dr. 171, 184, 204
Pietrocini, Jeremy 11, 335
Pink Pockets™, Post Mastectomy Drain Holders 214, 337
post-traumatic growth 21
Project LEAD 74

R

Radical Remission 21, 22, 336
Rath, Tom 28, 336
recurrence 35, 60, 91, 121, 155, 164, 170, 207
Red Devil 41
Relationship Building domain. *See* Gallup: domain: Relationship Building
Road to Recovery®. *See* American Cancer Society: Road to Recovery®

S

scalp hypothermia 206
scanxiety 163
Scott, Stuart 12, 335
second opinion 26, 52, 88, 89, 170
Sliekers, Stephanie 9
Smith, Dave 25
Sorenson, Susan 19
Stand Up to Cancer 61
Stanford University
    Cancer Mindset research 20
    Mind and Body Lab 19
Strategic Thinking domain. *See* Gallup: domain: Strategic Thinking
Sugg, Dr. 121, 171
survivorship 2, 21, 35, 88, 108, 159, 160, 174, 208, 211, 221, 222, 236, 240, 242, 319

T

Tedeschi, Richard, Dr. 21
Thich, Nhat Hanh 242, 337
Tumor Board 171
Turner, Kelly, Dr. 21, 22, 336

U

UIHC. *See* University of Iowa Health Care
University of Iowa Health Care 8, 167, 211, 212
University of Kansas School of Medicine 249

V

Valvano, Jim 98
V Foundation 12, 98, 335

W

Waterloo-Cedar Falls Courier 73
Winfrey, Oprah 251

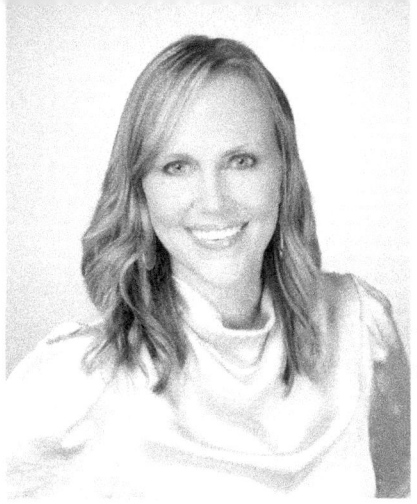

About the Author

Traci McCausland is the founder of Follow Your Strengths® and provides training and keynote speaking on leadership, employee engagement, and strengths-based development. She helps organizations develop leaders, build better teams, and create great places to work. Since becoming a Gallup-Certified Strengths Coach in 2014, she has trained more than 5,000 people in over 100 organizations worldwide.

In 2017, at the age of 39, Traci was diagnosed with breast cancer. This unexpected health challenge led her to reflect on concepts she teaches others—strengths, mindset, and authenticity. As the daughter of educators and a lifelong learner, she has remained engaged in the world of cancer survivorship. Traci now serves on the board of the American Cancer Society in Iowa and has traveled to Washington, D.C., to advocate for cancer survivors through the American Cancer Society Cancer Action Network and the National Breast Cancer Coalition. She believes that facing a cancer diagnosis is hard enough without additional barriers to quality care.

Traci holds degrees in management and organizations and counseling psychology from the University of Iowa and the University of Kansas. She lives in Waterloo, Iowa, with her husband, Kent, and their two children.

Feedback for *Surviving Cancer with Your Strengths* and Ways to Learn More

Share Your Praise
Did this book help you navigate a cancer journey or provide you support as a caregiver? Did it offer new insights into leveraging your strengths and mindset through the cancer experience? If so, we'd love it if you left a review with your favorite online retailer. A few minutes of your time could help other cancer survivors and caregivers discover this book during a challenging time.

Place a Bulk Order
Would you like to share *Surviving Cancer with Your Strengths* with your organization, institution, conference, event, or support group? We offer bulk discounts for orders of 10 or more copies to most locations. Please contact our team at publishing@followstrengths.com for more information.

Keep in Touch
For more about Traci's book, workshops, keynote speaking, and other offerings, please visit www.followyourstrengths.com. We provide customized services to a variety of audiences:
- Small businesses to large corporations
- Healthcare systems and cancer organizations
- Leadership and career development programs
- K-12 schools, students, staff, and administrators

Connect on Social Media
facebook.com/followyourstrengths
instagram.com/followyourstrengths
linkedin.com/in/traci-mccausland-speaker

www.ingramcontent.com/pod-product-compliance
Lightning Source LLC
Chambersburg PA
CBHW020531030426
42337CB00013B/807